Forever Linked

A Mother's Journey Through Twin to Twin Transfusion
Syndrome

Erin Bruch

This book is dedicated to all of the children and families touched by twin to twin transfusion syndrome, high risk pregnancy, or the loss of a pregnancy, infant, or child.

Contents

Contributors

Preface:

I am a mother of two boys, but they are no longer with me. I visit them weekly; I place flowers, whisper prayers, and sing songs to their headstone. The reason they are not here with me is due to a placental disease known as Twin-to-Twin Transfusion Syndrome. I know that until my boys were diagnosed with it, I never knew what it was or what it could do. This disease, Twin-to-Twin Transfusion Syndrome (TTTS), simply put, destroys families. It has the ability to take parents' simplest hopes and dreams and tear them apart within an instant. It can form an undesirable bond that can last through death. The destruction left in the wake of Twin-to-Twin Transfusion Syndrome is unimaginable, and different in every case. Even in the case that a child or children do survive the in utero disease, the family still copes with the voyage they endured. No one word can describe what a parent feels during the journey through Twin-to-Twin Transfusion Syndrome, and after the pregnancy has ended.

This book was written by moms willing to share their stories of success and devastation. 1 out of 4 pregnancies end in tragedy (not always by TTTS). If you know someone who is experiencing a loss, this book should give you an idea how to help your loved one through this difficult time.

Acknowledgments

I would like to acknowledge my husband, children, and family who have endured much over the course of writing this book. I know it was hard, but this book will help the newly diagnosed and their families deal and cope with TTTS and may help families cope with the loss of a baby. Your love and support is an unbelievable gift and I am truly thankful to have it each and every day.
Thank you to Toni Lopopolo, Literary Management and to Derrick Eisenhardt and his publishing house, Reliquary Press. You all helped so much in making this book into a reality. Thank you.

A special thanks to Dr. Daniele Focosi, MD; Dr. Ramen H. Chmait, M.D. - Director - Fetal Therapy Program; Dr. Julian De Lia, MD - Maternal-Fetal Medicine, Ob-Gyn; Fetal Hope Foundation; the Twin to Twin Transfusion Syndrome Foundation; Dr. Ramen Quintero - Professor and Director, Division of Maternal-Fetal Medicine, Director UM/Jackson Memorial Hospital Fetal Therapy Center, for allowing me to use your information to get the best information to be a part of this collaboration.

To Holly Bruce, Carolyn Bauder, Renee Walter RN., and Kim Bauder, you four have helped me face my darkest days; you pulled me from the ashes and helped me figure out what I was to do with my new life after the death of my twins.

And to my great friends who I think of almost every day, Rebecca Ruth Walker and Tonia Brundage-Amato, without you I never would have spoken up after my TTTS pregnancy. Thank you for helping me find my voice, you will be remembered.
Thank you to all of you.

Foreword

Parenthood is arguably the most important and exciting event in our lives as human beings. We have the opportunity and privilege to bring new life into the world and nurture our children to adulthood, experiencing the many joys, challenges, and occasional sorrows, with eventual acceptance of our children as individuals, all unique in their own right.

Pregnancy remains a singular event in the lives of women, entailing much emotional, physical and hormonal change, as well as fear, joy, and in most cases, eventual elation. As an obstetrician and perinatologist, I have had the honor and privilege of caring for many women with complicated pregnancies in my career. I have seen the strength of women, and their families, when faced with the unexpected loss of a child, born or unborn. There can be no more gut-wrenching experience in life than this.

Twin-twin transfusion syndrome (TTTS) is one such unanticipated event that, until recently, led to almost universal loss of both babies in an affected twin pregnancy. TTTS occurs when identical twin babies in utero share a single placenta. In about 15% of single placental twin pregnancies, the shared blood vessels in the placenta result in an unequal transfer of blood flow between the babies. The placenta sends more than normal amounts of blood, nutrients, and oxygen to the "recipient", and less than normal amounts to the "donor". Unfortunately, such a situation leads to complications for both babies in utero, and if left unattended, can lead, in the great majority of cases, to loss of both.

New understanding of fetal physiology and developments in high-resolution ultrasound technology have allowed us a previously unavailable opportunity to study fetal disease, and therefore to develop treatments for TTTS. Though the treatments are not yet perfected, you will read about some of them in this book. Rest assured, many of the brightest and best in medicine are making very frequent advances in treating TTTS. Today, in 2010, more than 70% of affected pregnancies experience a good outcome for one or both babies.

Beyond the overwhelming amount of information regarding treatment, the sudden and very personal drama of the pregnant woman, her spouse and family often goes without mention or appreciation. This book will bring you into the moment-to-moment thoughts, fears, hopes, joys and disappointments of families dealing with TTTS.

I think you will agree with me that the most profound lesson of this book is not so much the medical care now available in TTTS (though it is impressive and improving all the time), but the stories of the individual families, their abilities to rise to the challenge and deal with the constant emotional rollercoaster.

Indeed, I believe, the most significant lesson of this book is the perseverance and triumph of the human spirit in the face of adversity.

Albert P. Sarno, Jr, MD, MPH, Bethlehem, PA - June 2010

1
Why This Book Needed to be Written

I hope this book is the first of many to bring information to those who need it. More than likely you have never heard of Twin-to-Twin Transfusion Syndrome. I never received any information about it from my OB. Let's face it; our OB's cannot possibly have pamphlets for every type of complication that could arise in any pregnancy. I went to the bookstores and found nothing about TTTS. I had to rely on the Internet for shards of information regarding the disease, and knowing the Internet is not always 100% accurate, it was difficult choosing what I should pay heed, and what I shouldn't.

Once I saw the fetal surgical specialist, I received all the written information I could carry. Unfortunately, I had no solid way to inform my family members, no way to inform my friends. Even when I tried to tell people, some just thought I was making it up. TTTS is so evolved and case specific that even if someone could find the information regarding this disease, once they realized what I was facing, they would take a step back, be silent, and wait for news from me. I had no one to lean on. Even when I did try to put the "phone chain" into effect, the last person never received the correct information, which was even more frustrating. So much could take place so quickly; I lived hour-by-hour, day-by-day, and week-by-week. I still live this way, even years after my pregnancy ended.

If you have just found out that you are having twins, first and foremost CONGRATULATIONS! If you have just found out they are suffering from TTTS, I hope what happened to me will never happen to you. In these pages you will find actual accounts from mothers discussing their own pregnancies. If you are pregnant with twins suffering from TTTS, you will be asked many difficult questions by your doctor. Please know that this book is not meant to take the place of medical treatment. It is also not meant to scare you. With this disease, you must go to the doctor and seek out the best medical advice, so you can make the best decisions for you and your family. I myself had some information from my family doctor, the obstetrician, prenatal doctors, fetal surgeons, the NICU staff, and finally a personal grief counselor. You must make sure you feel comfortable with your doctors and with their advice. They deal with TTTS every day, and unfortunately now you will, too.

During this pregnancy you will also wish to tell your family members about what you are experiencing and what you need. You will gain comfort by educating others, and hope that maybe someone can come up with a cure and your children's lives will be saved. Personally, I know many people who, when told about TTTS, didn't believe it. If something was so badly wrong, they wondered, why didn't the pregnancy just end? Yes, every pregnancy does eventually end, but not all of them are happy endings. Many people cannot accept a baby's death. Many people I knew prior to my own TTTS pregnancy actually began to avoid me, because they could not comprehend the disease.

Even after months of being at home dealing with the loss, when I went back to work, I had to cope with my co-workers trying to enforce their own comfort levels when dealing with me and my boys.

You need to learn all you can about the disease. Create a positive support group. Please remember you did not cause TTTS. You did not do anything wrong in any way. You need to find friends and family members that will be a great sounding wall. No parent should be asked to kill one child to save the other. But each of us was. Some had no choice; others took a leap of faith and kept thinking "I am here for two babies, not just one."

Some women can't cope with TTTS, so they end the pregnancy before any other medical options are presented. This illustrates that each TTTS pregnancy is unique. Similar to how each person is different, each placenta is different, and each mother coping with this disease will make different decisions. That is key. You will need to search your own heart and figure out what you need to do for your family. Remember, no person has the right to judge you, EVER.

If you aren't pregnant, and just wish to take a moment to learn something new, these stories will give you a peek into a world that is not discussed, a world hidden under the rug. This is a horrible tragedy and needs to stop. When I finally returned to work, I was not allowed to have my sons' birth photos in my personal space; corporate said that my sons' pictures would "upset" my co-workers, even though they were from when my sons were alive. We need to step beyond our own comfort levels, and be selfless for our fellow man. We need to listen, learn, and gain an appreciation that we can be strong for our neighbors.

Your basic symptoms, all part of being pregnant, will be a part of this new journey, too. I started to show at week 12 with my twins, compared to week 26 with my daughter. I was drained, and tired all the time (which put a lot of stress on me at work), and I had extreme sciatic nerve pain with the twins. I was sick with my daughter, but never had morning sickness with the twins. Some of the mothers say that their morning sickness was worse with the twins than with their other babies. The thing with being pregnant is, all you can do is just compare notes and remember. Just because one woman felt a certain way during her pregnancy does not mean that you will feel the same way.

On average, a twin pregnancy has a much higher HCG rate then a singleton pregnancy. Keep in mind at the very start they look to have the same numbers for both.

Your levels can be completely different than the next person's. You will need to discuss any blood results with you doctor, to enable you to have the best care possible. During my twin pregnancy, my HCG results were at the top of the "normal range". So even though I knew I was pregnant, I didn't find out that I was having twins until the first ultrasound.

As you read through this book, you'll find I have taken a number of mothers' personal experiences and compiled them into sections. I never knew these women before this disease, I never spoke to them, or knew that this disease even existed.

Each person's experiences are told in their own words. For writing purposes, I may have omitted tangents, swear words, or even taken the liberty of organizing each woman's thoughts to keep the timeline moving.

Personally, I hope this book will bring comfort to those who are struggling, and let them know they are not alone. I particularly hope that this book will be able to grant a new mother, just diagnosed with TTTS, knowledge that I didn't have. Maybe we can learn from one another, to create different ways to treat TTTS' many symptoms, and to deal with its emotional side. Obviously, we need to put TTTS in the limelight to save our children's futures and get funding to help those who are now fighting for their lives. I know nothing can bring my boys back, but hopefully this book has the ability to help those who can be saved.

I know that during my TTTS pregnancy, I was terrified beyond belief, knowing that at any moment I needed to be ready to face the possibility of losing both of my children. Also, I needed to be prepared for the physical pain of the different procedures and surgeries. I needed to be able to cope with having a difficult time simply breathing when my children grew larger, along with the increasing amount of amniotic fluid levels. My only hope was to be able to hold them, and tell them how much I love them. I never let the pain show to anyone, only crying intensely when the twins were diagnosed with TTTS.

I believe that only through the pursuit of knowledge, can we overcome adversity. Each and every one of us has done just that. The only thing is, some of us have to live knowing our children died because the disease took too much. The lucky ones get to look at their child or children and be reminded, every day, what happened to them. We all wonder with TTTS, the "what if's", the "how come's", or my favorite, "why me's", but each of us was faced with this disease, and each of us carried our heads high through it. We have all learned more about ourselves then we ever knew, and found strength in others who have experienced with us.

So as you read this, I'm sure in many ways you will feel the roller coaster of emotions that each of us felt. You will have the amazing perspective to see what the mothers, whose twins have TTTS, go through. Even though you aren't hearing what the physicians are saying, hopefully you will be able to look at a pregnant woman and realize what she endures to bring her children into this world.

2
Before We Knew

BRUCH: I was on the pill, so we weren't really planning for more children. I had to deal with fertility treatments to conceive our daughter and wished that I could eventually get pregnant without medicinal help. We'd had two miscarriages before our living child. Losing the pregnancies was so difficult.

HADDIGAN: We were trying to have a baby for 4 to 5 years. We wanted a baby so badly.

SLICHTER: We were newlyweds. We were young, only 19. My husband is in the Marines. We were happy and just starting our new life together as a married couple. I moved away from my home, my family and friends to a new state where I didn't know anyone. Having children was not yet on our minds.

DICK: My husband, Trevor, and I met October 1, 2006. We knew it was love at first sight. We moved in together October 2, 2006, just a day after we met. It may seem crazy to some people, but to us, it just seemed natural.

CADLE: My husband, Ronnie, and I were talking about having more children, as we were already blessed with two children Radd (8), and Hannah (5). I said that it was now or never. We had moved 3 hours away from our family and friends because of Ronnie's work, so it was going to be a change with no family to help!

MARTIN: We were trying to get pregnant, but it was more of the "if it happened" kind of thing. I wanted another baby so badly. My 5 year old, from a previous relationship, was starting school. My husband and I just kind of clicked from the beginning, when we were dating, knowing that we wanted more children soon.

LIGHT: It's not like we tried or anything. I was 25 at the time, and it was a complete surprise.

CHRISTMAN-SCHARER: I had two wonderful sons from my first marriage, Tyler James, 8, and Alexander William, 6. I also had a son with Karl, Reid Morgan, who at the time was 7 months. He was a surprise for us.

MORGAN: We were actively trying for a year. It took us awhile to get pregnant which was surprising. I was 30 years old.

REBILAS: When we had our first son, we were ready for a sibling. We didn't start trying for a new baby until our son was nearing his first birthday. We tried to get pregnant for thirteen months! We suffered a miscarriage part way through.

Our doctor had urged us to give Clomid a try and we said no. I even joked with our obstetrician, I do NOT want twins! Too much work!

JELLEY: I was 23 years old and my husband, Cody, and I had been married for 3 years. We have a 3 year old son, Gareth, and had our baby girl, Eliza, in September. People kept saying we had the perfect family, and we said we would have another one when we were ready. Cody was leaving in February, for basic training in the Army National Guard, so we decided to take a chance that I wouldn't get pregnant before he left. Whenever we talked of the possibility, we would say it's ok if we have two babies close together. What's the big deal?

Cody left on Jan 30th, and it was really hard to say goodbye, knowing he was going to be gone for almost 5 months. We hadn't been apart for more than a few nights in about six years. We were told that he might be able to call, but it could be as long as months before he could. Thankfully, the fort where he ended up going allowed him to call every week.

BENNER: I was 20 when we were married on January 12, 2007. We thought we wanted to wait to have kids, but one day I woke up and decided it was time. We planned it perfectly. We only tried for one month.

HOPE: I felt that at 21, I was too young to have a baby. I was engaged to be married, and we lived 10 hours away from our families. I really thought it would be too hard for us to do it on our own. David, on the other hand, had wanted kids for ages; at 24 he felt it was time to start our family. After many hours up talking, I decided we would try. I would stop taking my pill and see what happened. I had spoken to so many people who had told me it would take months and months for me to fall pregnant. That was perfect! We would have time to adjust to the idea, as well as to start to saving and preparing. We told no one of our plan, as who knew when it would happen?

WRIGHT: My husband and I had been trying to get pregnant. We had both been married previously, and we each had children from our prior marriages, but we wanted one together - Yours, Mine, and Ours. I got pregnant right away, in May 2008. Unfortunately, I miscarried when I was only 5 weeks along. We were devastated. My husband is in the military and he ended up deploying at the end of the summer. He came home in December and we were told he'd have to deploy again in February. We only had two months to try. When the first month was unsuccessful, we used at- home ovulation predictor kits. I was 28 years old and my husband was 30.

DILLE: My husband and I were not trying to get pregnant. Jamie and I had been married for almost 5 years. We had a 6 year old named Tyler, and an 18 month old, Caylee. I had already come to terms with the fact that Caylee would be our last baby, because we were not really in a financial position to have more children.

BRAY: It was autumn 2008 and we were planning our wedding for September, 2009. I had just turned 28 and Gareth was 32. We had been together for 5 years and thought it was about time we finally made it official. We already had a 2 year old little boy, William, and had plans to try for another baby after the wedding.

OROSZ: My husband and I were trying to get pregnant with our second baby. Our first born son was about to turn 3. It took 2 months after getting off of the birth control pill. I was 26 years old when I found out.

FLETCHER: Before we knew we were pregnant with Ally and Abby, we had been trying for over a year. I had gone to my OB/Gyn and he put me on Clomid. He told me everything about the fertility drug and the percentage of twins. I love my doctor. I took Clomid for 2 months. I had stressed myself out so much over getting pregnant and finally just prayed about it, leav-

ing it in God's hands. With Austin, it had all happened so fast. No problems getting pregnant. I
would soon find out he was our easy pregnancy. He
was a day over due. No trouble with labor or delivery. I just wanted one more baby. I was 27 years old
when we started trying to get pregnant the second
time.

DOBBS: We knew we wanted to get pregnant, and
had had difficulties with our oldest. So we thought
nothing to the possibility of needing help this time.

WALLINGTON: Being a mother is what I dreamt of
when I was a child. Some people want to be a doctor
and some want to be star, but I just wanted to have
children of my own to love and nurture to become
good people.

Sean and I had finally conceived after 2 long
years of trying. We were so excited! I scheduled my
first doctor appointment at 8 weeks. Unfortunately, 3
days before my appointment I began to miscarry. On
September 12, 2004, we went in to the doctor's office,
only to be told I did indeed miscarry, and it was
twins. We were devastated, but shortly began to try
again.

BRUCE: My husband and I were actually still dating
at the time of conception. We were planning a beautiful fall wedding for October 2007. We had no idea
what was ahead of us.

3
The Disease

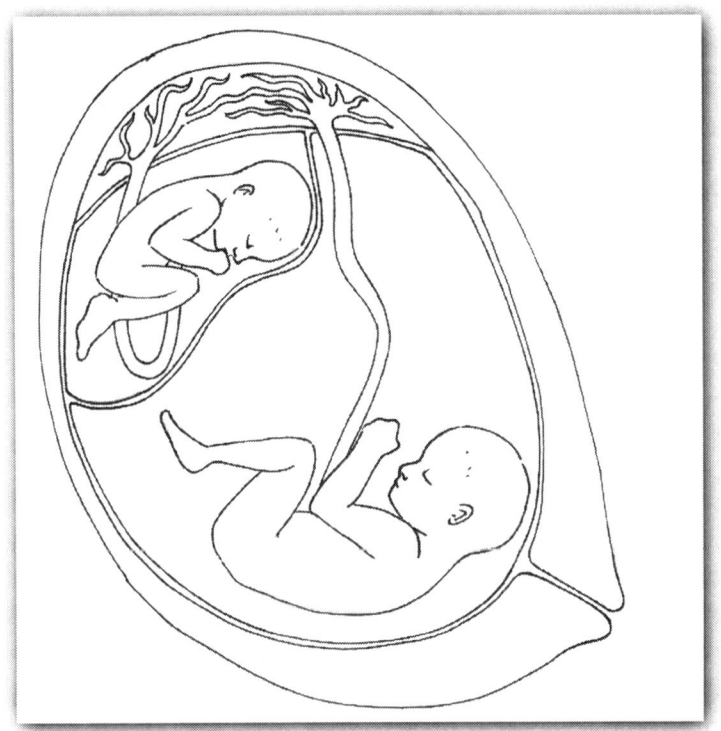

Mary Slaman-Forsythe of The TTTS Foundation explains that "twin to twin transfusion syndrome (TTTS) is a disease of the placenta. It affects identical twins during pregnancy when blood passes disproportionately from one baby to the other through connecting blood vessels within their shared placenta. One baby, the recipient twin, gets too much blood overloading his or her cardiovascular system, and may die from heart failure. The other baby, the donor twin, does not get enough blood and may die from severe anemia. The babies are normal. The abnormalities are in the placenta." Left untreated, 80-100% of the babies may pass away.

The cause of TTTS is attributed to unbalanced flow of blood through vascular channels that connect the circulatory systems of each twin via the common placenta. The shunting of blood through the vascular communications leads to a net flow of blood from one twin (the donor) to the other twin (the recipient). The donor twin develops oligohydramnios (low amniotic fluid) and poor fetal growth, while the recipient twin develops polyhydramnios (excess amniotic fluid), heart failure, and hydrops. If left untreated, the pregnancy may be lost due to lack of blood getting to the smaller twin, fluid overload and heart failure in the larger twin, and/or preterm (early) labor leading to miscarriage of the entire pregnancy. (*Courtesy of the Fetal Hope Foundation*)

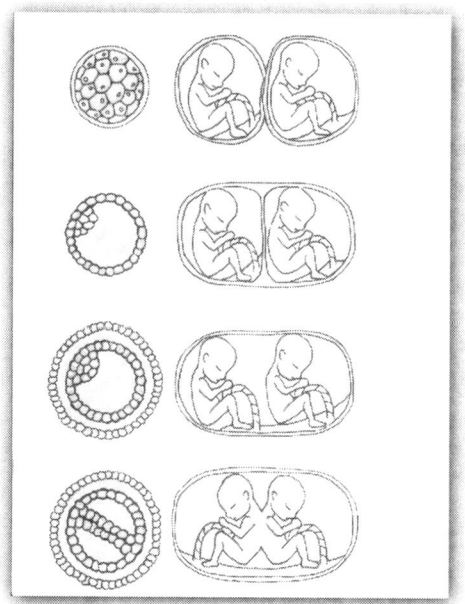

The timing of the separation of the egg is crucial in a TTTS case. As you can see from this diagram, days 4 to 13are critical in the development of TTTS.

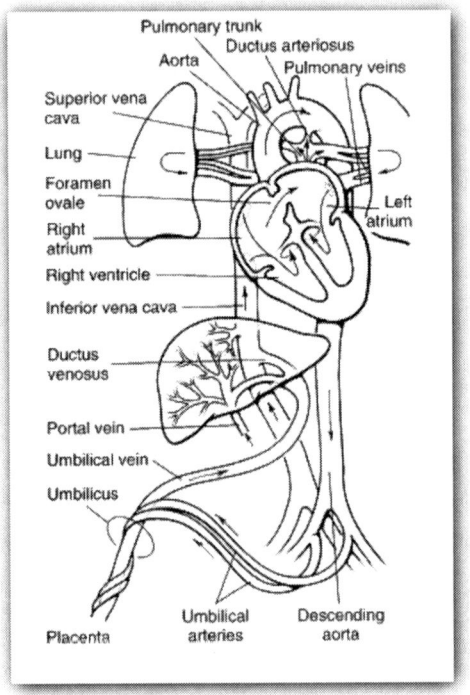

Pulmonary trunk
Ductus arteriosus
Aorta
Pulmonary veins
Superior vena cava
Lung
Foramen ovale
Right atrium
Left atrium
Right ventricle
Inferior vena cava
Ductus venosus
Portal vein
Umbilical vein
Umbilicus
Placenta
Umbilical arteries
Descending aorta

In: Molecular Medicine©. Copyright, Daniele Focosi. 2001-2005. Available at http://www.mm.interhealth.info: Educational Materials:Physiology of Adult HomoSapiens. Accessed 1/11.

Here is a diagram of a fetal circulatory system. This diagram will help you to understand where certain important vessels and connections lie in your children's bodies. This way when the doctors start stating how your TTTS case is advancing, you will be able to understand the severity of the case, which will allow you to make the most informed decision, not only for your children, but your future.

The arteries and veins are the main focus of finding a cure. These simple structures are found in every placenta. The underlying problem of TTTS is the placement of them. The connections can be a direct link, such as an artery to artery; an artery to a vein; veins to arteries; or a complex connection, such as multiple arteries to a vein. Remember that arteries carry oxygenated blood cells, and veins carry used

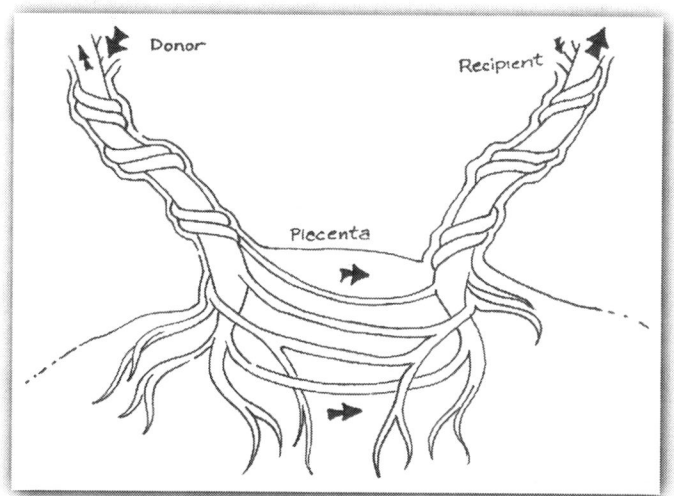

blood that is on the way to being re-oxygenated. The issue is, when you have "used" blood from one twin directly passing directly to the second, the second then gets fewer nutrients and develops on a smaller scale.

Please keep in mind that just because a twin is smaller in size, it does not automatically make him/her disabled. My boys differed by 40% at birth, but both had muscle tone, both could hold your finger, both could move, and both reacted to my voice. The only way for disability to occur is if one or the other does not get enough oxygen. Also the more prematurely a baby is born, the higher chance of learning disabilities such as ADD, ADHD, Autism, or other conditions. Please speak with your doctor to weigh each medical option and find the right plan for your specific case.

When I was first diagnosed with TTTS, the doctor explained what he found in my ultrasound that made him arrive at the diagnosis.

1) Monochorionicity, a discrepancy in amniotic fluid between the amniotic sacs with polyhydraminos of one twin (largest vertical pocket greater than 8 cm) and oligohydraminos of the other (largest vertical pocket less than 2 cm)
2) Discrepancy in size of the umbilical cords
3) Cardiac dysfunction in the polyhydramniotic twin
4) Abnormal umbilical artery or ductus venosus (Doppler velocimetry)
5) Significant growth discordance (often greater than 20 percent)

He then explained another type of staging that depending on the severity would increase as the pregnancy prolonged.

Quintero Staging System for Twin-Twin Transfusion
Syndrome:

1) Stage I: polyhydraminos in the recipient, severe oligohydraminos in donor but urine visible within the donor's bladder
2) Stage II: polyhydraminos in the recipient, a
   "stuck" donor, urine not visible within the donor's bladder
3) Stage III: polyhydraminos and oligohydraminos as well as critically abnormal Doppler's (at
   least one of: absent or reverse end diastolic
   flow in the umbilical artery, reverse flow in the
   ductus venosus or pulsate umbilical venous
   flow) with or without urine visible within the
   donor's bladder
4) Stage IV: presence of ascites or frank hydrops
   (fluid collection in two or more cavities) in either donor or recipient
5) Stage V: demise of either fetus.

This staging system is descriptive. The risk of fetal death and neurological issues increases pro-
gressively on the Quintero Stage.

There are a few ways to treat TTTS. Depending on your case, your doctor will help you choose
which is best. My doctor became amazed by what I
began to understand and learn during my own TTTS
pregnancy. Even to this day, I can still remember the
doctors informing me of treatment options and how
they determine the severity of TTTS in each patient.

Below are the different treatment options for TTTS. This will give you an idea of what the doctors will say once you see them. They will evaluate your case and make recommendations for your family. Please keep in mind that regardless of your treatment and its outcome, you will have to make peace with whatever decision you make.

According to Ramen H. Chmait, M.D. Director, Fetal Therapy Program of Maternal-Fetal Medicine, Ob-Gyn (Keck School of Medicine, University of Southern California) the different treatment options offered to a family facing twin to twin transfusion syndrome are:

1. Expectant Management: In general, if no treatment is instituted during the pregnancy, there is an almost 100% risk of pregnancy loss. There are two main reasons for this. First, the excessive amount of amniotic fluid that develops in the sac of the recipient twin causes severe distension of the womb, contractions, and miscarriage or extreme premature birth. Second, the stress of the disease can result in the death of one twin in the womb. Because the livelihoods of the twins are linked together by the blood vessels that they share, the death of one twin in the womb can result in 30% chance of brain damage or death to the co-twin.

2. Termination: A second option that a family can choose is to terminate the entire pregnancy. This option is considered because of the high risks associated with TTTS, available treatments of TTTS, and the risk of premature births. Babies that are born too early have increased risk of brain injury, lung problems, gut problems, etc. Also, the stress of the high-risk pregnancy can be overwhelming, given that both babies will not survive. By terminating

the pregnancy, the parents can start the grieving process and try to move on with their lives.

3. Serial amniocentesis is a procedure that is used periodically to relieve the recipient twin of the excess accumulation of amniotic fluid. For this procedure, a needle is used to enter the mother's uterus and the recipient twin's amniotic sac, which is then drained of fluid. By decreasing the amount of water in the recipient twin's sac, the amount of distension of the womb is decreased, thereby lessening the chances of delivering the babies too early. For Quintero Stage I and II TTTS, there is an approximately 85% chance that at least one baby will survive, and a 50% chance that both babies will survive. For Stage III and IV TTTS, there is about a 50% chance of at least one twin survivor, and a 33% chance for both to survive. The risk of long term brain injury is higher in the advanced stages, with a 25% risk of neurologic impairment.

4. Endoscopic laser surgery is a procedure in which a small puncture is made in the mother's abdomen and a fetoscope is inserted into the amniotic cavity. This allows the surgeon to look into the uterus and use a laser to occlude all the vascular communications between the twins. If all of the connecting blood vessels are successfully laser ablated, then the TTTS is essentially cured. We discovered an approximately 90% chance of survival of at least one twin and a 70% chance of survival of both twins. Regardless of the severity of the disease, there is an approximately 5% risk of neurologic impairment.

5. Amniotic Septostomy is a procedure in which a needle is inserted into the mother's abdomen, and the membrane between the two twins is punctured to cause artificial equilibration of amniotic fluid between the two sacs. This option is of historical

interest only. There is no role for this procedure in the contemporary treatment of TTTS.

    6. <u>Umbilical cord ligation</u> (tying of the umbilical cord) is performed endoscopically (through a small puncture in the mother's abdomen) when one twin is severely compromised. Many centers have stopped offering cord ligation for the treatment of TTTS. First, this approach results in the obligate demise of one twin. In other words, that baby is sacrificed for the sake of the other twin. However, we have found that even "gravely sick" fetuses can recover normally after laser surgery, making that a far more attractive option. Second, both the calibre of the instruments used and the surgical risks are similar to that of endoscopic laser surgery. Therefore, ligation offers neither decreased risk nor better outcome than laser surgery. If a center suggests ligation and you are uncomfortable with this, seek a second opinion at another center.

In conversation with Dr. Julian De Lia MD., I learned that the mother's diet will also have a huge impact on the outcome of the pregnancy. The mother should sip high protein shakes slowly during the day and eat a high caloric diet during her pregnancy.

Each and every Twin-to-Twin Transfusion Syndrome pregnancy is unique. It never presents itself the same way twice. After each TTTS pregnancy ends, specialists look at the placenta closely to learn new information. This is very important, especially if endoscopic laser surgery was performed. These specialists can do "injection studies" to see if there are any remaining patent anastomoses (open blood vessel connections between the twins). Unfortunately, not everyone can send their placenta to the appropriate researchers, so much information is lost every day. My own placenta looked like a 36-week, when it was only 24 weeks. It had other rare abnormalities, but we will not fully know their cause, or the effect that they had, until more cases are found that have these abnormalities.

Terrified, Dramatic, Astounded, Lectured , Inferior, Overprotected, Scared, Threatened, Vulnerable, Unsafe, Robbed, Cheated, Uninformed, Unsupported, Powerless, Pressured, Restricted, Bullied, Controlled, Imprisoned, Inhibited and Forced (and the list goes on), are all things you can feel during a TTTS pregnancy. Each family needs to develop a support group. The Internet was a great place to discover people who could help me understand not only what was happening to my babies, but to my own health, and how that was affecting my family. Emotionally, this is a horrific disease, and as a personal note, I would recommend seeing a counselor to help release the feelings that might otherwise increase a mother's stress.

4
Finding Out We Were Pregnant

BRUCH: I had the feeling I was pregnant, but was unsure. I never asked what the HCG results were. I figured that after being through infertility treatments with my previous pregnancy, if the doctor wasn't alarmed by the results, I shouldn't be either.

HADDIGAN: A home pregnancy test was finally positive!

SLICHTER: It happened quickly, very soon after I had moved, in September of 2005. I didn't realize it at first as I had never been pregnant before and didn't really know what to expect. I had missed my period, but didn't really think much of it. I remember walking up the stairs and I could just feel my lower stomach was tighter. That is when I thought I had to be pregnant. I went to the store and picked up a home pregnancy test and waited until the next morning. As I waited for the lines to change, I had a wave of emotions come over me. I was nervous, scared, and excited. Sure enough, there were two pink lines on it. We were shocked and scared to say the least, but we were very happy. I went to the doctor's office to confirm and a few days later I got the call that indeed I was pregnant.

DICK: A few months after we got together, we found out we were pregnant. This was December 2006. It all happened so fast. I was excited, nervous, happy, and scared all at the same time. I was only 18, but I knew I would be a great mom. From the moment we took the test, I couldn't wait for my baby to be born. I remember sitting in our room, waiting for the results to come through on the test. When it came back "pregnant", I just looked at my (now) husband, and smiled.

CADLE: Right after we moved, we got pregnant (instantly). I was at work and had realized that my work clothes were not fitting right. They were really snug, which was really weird because I worked out every day. So I went to the store and brought 2 things: a pregnancy test and a box of feminine products. I remember the cashier looking at me funny and I told her "Well it's one or the other!" I went back to work, took the test, and brought it out to show my co-worker in disbelief! I really did not think I was going to be pregnant that fast. I had only been trying for a few weeks. The lines were so blue that I was amazed. With Radd and Hannah I had to buy tons of tests, and never got two bright blue lines. There was always one bright and one lighter line. A few days later I made an appointment because I was cramping (contraction cramping). Everyone said that there was no way I was contracting, but I told them that I was and that it was very odd.

MARTIN: It all started in April when I felt that my breasts were really sore, and then four tests later my assumption proved correct. This was great -- my husband's first, and a new hope to actually have another baby, which I wanted so badly. The time line was perfect. I wanted this more than anything for my birthday which had JUST passed. My husband was ecstatic!! He called everyone in his family as soon as we found out. It was hard for him to believe that his hopes and wishes were finally coming true. After many failed attempts and prayers, we were finally pregnant.

TUMMERS: We had a little "incident" that I referred to, while being repeatedly interviewed by medical students during my stay in the hospital, as "the proof why they tell you in sex education class to always have a back-up method". I knew the chances were pretty good that I would get pregnant, but was still pretty surprised when the nurse beamed at me and said, "It's most definitely positive!" I felt good about this change of plans, an opportunity to cherish all those final moments and maybe the motivation to get our lives on track. I was about 5.5 weeks along at this point.

LIGHT: Rob and I found out we were going to be parents on November 13th, 2007. Aside from the usual dizziness and morning sickness associated with the first few months, everything seemed to be going alright. Little did we know…

CHRISTMAN-SCHARER: Karl and I were only dating 3 months when I found out I was pregnant with Reid, and now I was pregnant again?! It was a moment I won't soon forget.

MORGAN: We took two home pregnancy tests and they came back positive. My husband's reaction was, in a word, excited. He had wanted children for a long time. No worries at all. Not a single worrisome thought.

REBILAS: We found out on New Year's Day! I KNEW I was pregnant! I was only two weeks along, but I knew! When I took the test and it was purple right away, I looked at my husband and said, "We're pregnant, and I think it's twins!" I am sure there is no medical proof for that, but since I was still two weeks early for my cycle and already testing positive, it was my first clue. Later that night, I had the first of many dreams that hinted twins were in our future.

JELLEY: I was already feeling tired and a little sick. I decided to joke around about it so if I was pregnant no one would be in shock. Of course when I said I was feeling sick, I would get, "Well the flu is going around.", and when I was tired, "Well you did have a long day." My baby hadn't been nursing very well and it really made me wonder if something was going on.

About a week after Cody had left, I took Eliza to the doctor for a well-child checkup. She hadn't gained any weight in a month and as we were discussing that, I told the doctor she wasn't nursing very well and that I was feeling pregnant. The doctor said, "Oh, do you want to pee real fast?" I almost said no. I really didn't want to know, because I couldn't tell anyone until my husband called, and who knew when that would be? And then I would get everyone judging me for getting pregnant, since my baby was only 5 months old! But I decided I might as well take a test. It would probably be negative and then I could brush off being sick, etc. After a little ordeal, the medical assistant came in and said, "It's positive!" She had been the one to tell me that almost exactly one year before.

I left the office a little in shock; I think I was even shaking. I called my mom and told her, "You can't tell anyone but... I'm pregnant." My mom is also a midwife and had delivered both my babies.

BENNER: It was Friday, September 7th, 2007, when I went out and bought a pregnancy test. I came home and took it. It was positive. I thought that I was a day late, but realized that I was actually a week late, because of how the month had fallen. That night after I got off work, I showed my husband, Jacob, the test. He responded with "Is this really your pee?" I said yes - duh. We stayed up all night thinking, talking and just loving it. The next morning I took another to be sure. Still positive. We were so very sure it would take months. But nope, God gave us a gift, and we were going to take very good care of it. On Tuesday, September 11, it was confirmed at a clinic. I was about 5 1/2 weeks pregnant. We were so excited.

HOPE: I was sitting in our kitchen one night, talking to David as he was cooking us dinner, and it is very hard to describe the feeling I had, kind of like butterflies across my tummy. It was unusual, something I had never felt before, and I instantly knew I was pregnant. I turned and said to David, "I'm pregnant." I had a home test in the bathroom and we thought about doing that, but I was still 3 days from my period and I thought it would be a waste. In the end I couldn't help myself; I did it and it was positive. We were both so excited. I, more so on the outside. On the inside, I was freaking out, it had only been 3 months since I stopped taking my pill. It wasn't supposed to happen this fast. Immediately we phoned both of our parents. David's parents were ecstatic, mine quite the opposite. They felt I was too young, and financially it would be a huge struggle. Over time they accepted and became happy with my news.

WRIGHT: I found out four days before my husband deployed that I was pregnant. I ended up taking six different tests just to make sure. My husband and I were ecstatic! He was supposed to be deployed for six months. It was exciting that as soon as he'd get home we would be having a baby.

DILLE: I could tell that I was pregnant by some physical symptoms that I had. They began at the time that I should have started my cycle. I bought a HPT to confirm it and it turned out positive. I was in shock and thought maybe the test was wrong because it wasn't a name brand, so I went back to the store and got another double pack. I took both of those over the next couple of hours and they both came back positive as well. Even though I felt the physical symptoms, I was still in shock since we weren't trying to get pregnant. It took 2 years of trying with my then 18 month old, so I never thought we would get pregnant again without even trying. My husband was just as surprised as I, but was supportive and happy about having another baby. I was neither worried nor relieved when I found out that I was pregnant. I was just very surprised, and happy with the thought of having another baby.

BRAY: October came, and I was a few days late with my period. I had that sick, bloated feeling for a few days but hadn't really thought anything of it. It suddenly hit me. I was pregnant! I knew it!

I didn't say anything to Gareth. I went out and bought a test, sat on the toilet, and waited for the results. Two very long minutes later.....POSITIVE! I ran downstairs and showed Gareth. He almost fell off of the chair. Along with William, Gareth had 2 daughters from a previous marriage, so to say he was shocked is a bit of an understatement. It was such an odd feeling. I was so pleased that I was pregnant, yet disappointed in myself for being so careless (we had booked our wedding and everyone was looking forward to it). We put a hold on the wedding plans and started getting excited about the thought of having a new little bundle of joy to look after.

OROSZ: I took a pregnancy test mainly because we were trying. I thought for sure it would come back negative. My husband was very happy we conceived, since we were trying. We felt very relieved. Now the waiting began.

FLETCHER: The day we found out we were pregnant was the last of November. I remember taking a ton of pregnancy tests because I could not believe it had finally happened. I remember calling my husband at work. He was super excited, as were Austin and I. I just remember being so excited. I wanted to shout it from the rooftops. Austin was telling everyone he was going to have a little sister. He wanted to name her "Rileybug", like his cousin.

I told him we couldn't name her Riley because we already had a Riley in our family. So he thought for a few minutes, and looked at me. Then he said, "What about Ally-bug?" I was like, "Sure, that sounds like a great name." He was only 4 at the time. He is mature beyond his years. I can remember telling our families. It was such a happy time in our lives.

DOBBS: It's May 26, 2005, and my husband and I are on our way to the OBGYN's office to get the results of the testing to determine why I am not having a period. We enter the examination room and it seems like forever until the doctor comes in. We discuss our options and decide that I will take pills to help me ovulate, after a failed insemination in late November of 2004. The doctor says before we can receive the pills she will have to do a pregnancy test. As the doctor leaves the room to perform the test, Michael looks at me and says "Is that what you want to do?" I say, "It took us four years to get pregnant with our daughter, Kendra, so there is no way we are pregnant." The doctor comes back into the room and says, "Guess what? You are pregnant."

I soon make an appointment with Dr. P., my OBGYN, and an ultrasound confirms that I am pregnant. He then says to my husband and I that we need to come back in two weeks for another ultrasound. We think nothing of this and go home to tell our parents I am expecting again.

WALLINGTON: In February 2005, we found out that I was pregnant again.

BRUCE: Since we had just been married on March 26, 2007, we had to wait until I was covered under my husband's medical insurance before visiting the doctor. We finally made it to my OB on April 13th. The doctor had blood drawn and started me on prenatal vitamins. They also scheduled my first ultrasound for the following Friday. I was showing already, and had to break out my maternity jeans from my first pregnancy (with my son). My mother-in-law teased me about my early belly bump and said that I was carrying twins. I just laughed at her and told her that I gained a lot of weight with my first, and everyone always told me that you show faster with your second, so that's probably what it was.

5
Normal Doctor's Appointments

BRUCH: I was showing, and was concerned by that, but just brushed off my size. This was my second pregnancy after all. I thought of twins, but what were the odds? I was just so happy this was a "normal", non- high-risk pregnancy. The NP didn't think much at this point. She figured this being my second pregnancy was the reason I was bigger. I asked for an ultrasound, but she wouldn't do one. She made me feel like I was a crazy woman.

HADDIGAN: At week 6 during the pregnancy, I was having lower abdominal pain. My OB appointment wasn't for another 2 weeks, so they recommended that I go to my family doctor. Our family doctor said there was no reason that the pregnancy would be causing my pain. She recommended that I take it easy and sent me home.

DICK: I went to my regular doctor to get the pregnancy test confirmed, considering we only took a store bought test. The test confirmed that I was indeed pregnant. My doctor said she wanted to see me back in a month! I went back a month later and she checked for the heartbeat with a sonogram. There was ONE solid, steady heartbeat. My husband and I were thrilled. Now, all we had to wait for was to find out the sex!

CADLE: During week 7, I went in and the doctor did a pelvic sonogram and said that the baby was where it was supposed to be, and that I would have to come back. Just to let you know, the more time goes by, the more I remember. I have not told anyone this, but I promise at that sonogram, I saw more than one baby. I just didn't think anything about it since I had no idea what I was seeing. I was just relieved that everything was okay. I had gained about 6 pounds and was not even eating that much. This pregnancy was crazy as I hurt all the time.

During week 10, I got all of my lab slips and told my nurse that I was short of breath. When she took my blood pressure, it was 122/62, and she said that the top number was high, but I was fine. I told her that I needed to get my tooth fixed, since I had chipped it on some beef jerky! She asked my doc and he gave the okay. The next day I went to the dentist, and while I was lying there, I had a really weird feeling in my belly. The dentist asked if I was ok, and I told her yes, but she told me to call my doctor and tell him what had happened. My doctor told me to drink some water and put my feet up, so I did. At this point I was very nauseous and felt worse than before. My friends would say, "You're not that young anymore and your body has changed", because I was morning sickness free with Radd and Hannah! I would tell people, "Don't wait until you get older to have kids, because it is way different." I had to stop cooking because the smells made me sick. I had morning sickness all day, every day, for weeks.

During week 12, I was at work, and my co-worker and I were going to lunch. I was walking down the sidewalk and I had this sharp pain. It was bad enough that I grabbed my belly and leaned over a little. My co-worker asked if I was okay. I said yeah and continued to lunch. When we got back, I told her to look at and feel my belly. It was hard and big. I mentioned that I was having contractions and was freaking out a little. So I called my so- called doctor, and he said his famous line: "Drink some water and put your feet up." "Whatever," I thought, but I did what he said. Ronnie and our children were kind of suffering because I was tired, sick and hurting. It was so hard for them, but we were all very happy and excited. Radd and Hannah always saw Daddy kiss Mommy's belly. They picked up on this, and would come talk to their baby brother or sister.

During week 14, I was up 12 pounds and once again I told the nurse the same thing as last time - I was short of breath. My B.P. was 138/82 and still there was no concern. I walked like I was 8 months pregnant, and it hurt. I knew that there was something wrong but I did not know what!

During week 15, I recall a lady at the store I stopped at every morning said, "Wow! You are getting big. How far along are you now?" I said almost 16 weeks. She could not believe it. She thought that I was at least 6 months. I was big.

MARTIN: We had an ultrasound on the first visit, since my last 2 pregnancies resulted in miscarriage around the 6th week. We saw a heartbeat and we were okay. Everything had checked out just fine. The doctor, at the time, seemed to be an outstanding man. He really seemed to care, or at least so we thought, since he took the time to reassure us that we were okay. He took his time on the ultrasound, and completely understood our worries. I felt very safe in his care.

TUMMERS: As soon as I knew I was pregnant, I called the midwife from my last pregnancy. My first appointment with her was in week 9. A friend from

work had experienced a horrible chromosomal abnormality in her pregnancy a few months before, so
we decided that we'd like to do the IPS screening this
time. I felt very different with this pregnancy than
with the boys, and was certain it was a girl.

LIGHT: We had one "normal" doctor appointment.
He was very positive and covered the basics: weight
gain, blood pressure, depression and morning sickness. Nothing about being high-risk was ever stated.

MORGAN: During my first doctor's appointment,
she detected one heartbeat – but didn't know to look
for two. We still assumed that it was a singleton
pregnancy. She reminded me to take my pre-natal vitamins…very simple, laid back appointment. She
scheduled me for an ultrasound at Phoenix Perinatal;
she did not have an ultrasound machine in her office.

REBILAS: I told my doctors it was twins at my week
8 appointment and they didn't believe me. They assured me I was too small (Never heard that before, I
can assure you!). I told them that I truly felt two little
rushes in my stomach. At my week 12 appointment, I
told the doctor again that I really felt it was twins, but
he didn't believe me and wouldn't check for another
heartbeat. I just shrugged it off at this point; they
were my doctors, surely they knew more than I did!

HOPE: Later, I had my first visit with my GP. She
was thrilled and sent me for all the normal tests. We
discussed how my lifestyle was to change, which vitamins I should be taking, and things I should be
starting to think about. By this stage I was so excited,
and then even more so when all my test results returned normal. We were given a referral for a week
12 ultrasound and decided to use an obstetrician in

the next town. Around week 10, we did the 10 hour drive home to see family and started buying little bits and pieces for our new baby. I was extremely sick; my morning sickness lasted 13 hours a day and would come on suddenly. I don't think I have ever thrown up as much in my whole entire life. But all in all, things were going smoothly and we were all very happy.

WRIGHT: I only had one regular visit with my OB (at ten weeks) before I was sent to a perinatologist. The OB congratulated me on my twins and briefly went over the risks that are associated with identical twins. Reviewing the ultrasound pictures the ER had sent, my OB thought that the twins might be mono-chorionic, mono-amniotic. They could not see the dividing membrane between my babies.

DILLE: My very first doctor appointment was for an ultrasound. I had some spotting at 5 ½ weeks and thought maybe I had miscarried. I continued feeling strange for a week after the spotting, so my doctor suggested I come in for a scan right at 7 weeks. At that point I would be far enough along to hear a heartbeat. It was there that I found out about the twins. From week 7 until our diagnosis at week 19, all of our appointments were completely normal and routine. I went in and got to hear the heartbeats and most times had a quick ultrasound, to check on the babies. I was told at one of these appointments that it looked like we had monochorionic, diamnionic twins, which meant that they were identical twins who shared a placenta but each had their own amniotic sacs. I did not go through the normal pregnancy testing as the results would be altered because of the 2 babies.

BRAY: We made an appointment with the doctor, who referred us to our local antenatal clinic. He stated that as we had no problems with our previous pregnancy, our care would be midwife led. The midwife came to visit us at home at the end of October, and we booked our first ultrasound scan for December. I had no real problems at this point. I suffered the usual morning sickness and headaches, but noticed nothing out of the ordinary. It seemed that everything was going to be textbook, just like the first pregnancy.

OROSZ: I started going to my normal gynecologist, who had delivered my first son. My friend is an ultrasound tech; she scanned me so I could see the heartbeat, and we saw what she thought was two. I joked with her, asking, "There's only one in there, right?" So I called my doctor and had her schedule an ultrasound to confirm, and at 7 weeks, sure enough, it was TWINS.

6
O My Goodness TWINS or MORE!

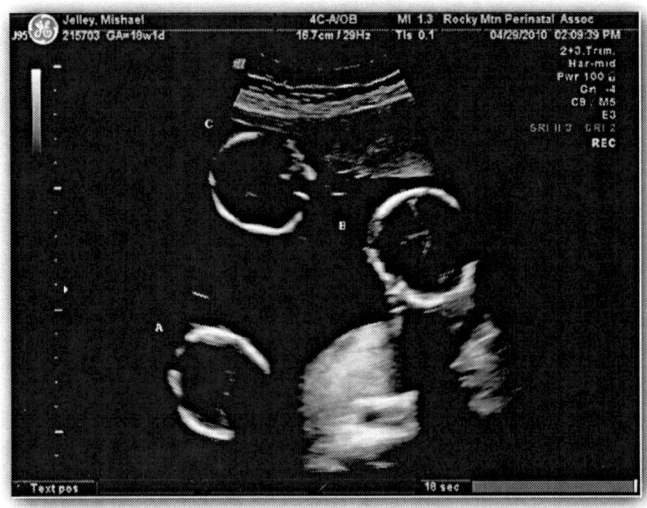

<u>BRUCH:</u> At this point we were 13 weeks along. I couldn't believe it, I was huge! The ultrasound technician asked, "How are you doing?"

I replied happily, "I am just so relieved that I can enjoy this time, that this is not a high risk pregnancy." She looked at me and said, "You don't know?" I said, "Know what?" She said, "You are having twins!"

I was in shock for a good hour; could I handle two babies? But I wanted them with all my heart, and wished for them to be healthy. My aunt had identical twins; if she could do it, so could I! They mentioned that I would be watched, and that we needed to make sure that the issues that come from twin pregnancy were identified early. I was just floored.

HADDIGAN: I remember it so well. It was during week 8, our first OB appointment. To confirm how far along the pregnancy was, my ob did an ultrasound. The tech was seeing something that she couldn't explain, and left to get the doctor to look at it. They discussed what they were seeing, and finally told us that there were two heartbeats. No question. The doctor went on to tell us of all the problems that come along with a twin pregnancy. One of which was TTTS. We discounted it, figuring that the odds of identicals were so small and then the odds of having TTTS, too -- we had nothing to worry about. For the next 6 weeks I had severe pain in my stomach, but the doctor always sent me home. He said, "There is nothing to worry about."

SLICHTER: After the confirmed pregnancy test with my doctor, I scheduled a prenatal appointment. It was in about two weeks. I had already told most of my family and friends at that time, and a lot of them teased me about being pregnant with twins. Even my mother had a strange feeling that it was twins, but I was skeptical. I went to the doctor's office as nervous as could be. I filled out the paperwork, and they took the usual vitals. I knew I was going to be getting an ultrasound, and that was what I was most looking forward to. As the doctor set everything up, I was laying there with loads going on in my mind. The machine came on, and the doctor said, "OK there's the baby, and it has a nice strong heartbeat and it is about eleven weeks along." I was so happy and relieved. Then all of a sudden he said, "Wait a minute, there are two." I did a double take, and asked him, "What? Really?" We were so happy. The look on my husband's face was happiness, but I could see a little bit of nervousness as well. The doctor was shocked, too.

He even called in some of his doctor and nurse buddies to come see the twins. Since it was a twin pregnancy, considered high risk, my general practitioner was uncomfortable overseeing this pregnancy, so he sent me across the hall to better obstetricians with better machines and equipment. I went, and was taken immediately to get another ultrasound. The tech noticed right away that something was wrong-- a cystic hygroma on one twin's neck. They were going to send me to doctor that was better trained in high risk matters. It was silent as I cried and cried the whole way home.

DICK: Well, April 17, 2007, I was sent for an ultrasound, and the ultrasound tech says "You're having a girl... wait, hold on a sec.... there's two! You're having identical twin girls!" I was ecstatic! "You mean to tell me no one told you that you were having twins?!" she said. I told her I had no idea. I couldn't believe it. How could they miss another baby? Regardless, I was thrilled and couldn't wait to phone and tell my husband. He was expecting one little boy, but he was about to get surprised with two baby girls! He was so happy and kept telling me, "I told you that you were getting too big to be having just one!" At that point, I hadn't even heard of TTTS. I just knew that I was going to have two beautiful baby girls, and that I was going to do everything possible to make sure they were healthy.

CADLE: During week 16, December 22, 2005, Ronnie and I went for our first sonogram. We were so excited. We had decided to find out the sex, but keep it a secret from family and friends! It hurt so badly to lie down. My stomach was so tight, and I remember just how badly it hurt! A few weeks before, one of my sisters had said we were having twins because I was so big. As the tech scanned my belly, there he/she was, beautiful and perfect. She started measuring. Seeing the heartbeat was always a relief. She asked how far along I was again, and I told her almost 17 weeks. She said the baby looked fine. Then she was checking other things and before we could tell her we wanted to know the sex, there was another baby! What?! I looked up at Ronnie, and he had this smile and did this shake thing with his head. We were speechless. She measured baby B then, and he was smaller – about 15 weeks. Still, he/she looked perfect. Once again, before we could find out what the sexes were, there was what looked to be another baby... Oh my goodness! 3 babies!

We had no time to be happy. The tech left the room to get the doctor. An inhumane person came in and said that baby C had no heartbeat and was only developed 10 weeks. I did not understand. Here is what the impression paper says:

1. Three intrauterine fetuses.

2. Est. fetal age of Fetus A: 16wks and 3 days EDC 06-05-06

3. Est. fetal weight of Fetus A: 158 grams

4. Est. fetal age of Fetus B: 15wks. 1 day EDC 06-14-06

5. Est. fetal weight of Fetus B: 112 grams

6. The third fetus appears to be deformed, with no heart activity. (Fetus C was definitely deformed and no measurements could be obtained. No heart activity was demonstrated in Fetus C. The amount of amniotic fluids appears to be increased. I believe that at

least two placentas are present.)

Our lives were forever changed in a matter of minutes. We had no idea what to do, what to say, but to cry. The dumb doctor said that I needed to be strong for the two healthy babies that were growing inside of me. I asked, "What we do now?" He replied, "No rush. After the holidays, call your doctor for further instructions.", and said that my body would take care of baby C. He also had the nerve to tell me that sometimes God makes mistakes. "Huh?" I replied, "No, if there is one thing that I know for sure, it's that God is perfect and He makes no mistakes!" I went into the bathroom and lost it. I walked out and took the sonogram picture of baby A. That's all I got that day; they gave me no pictures, none. I had to basically steal the one I did get. We left. I called one of my sisters and tried to tell her, but was so hysterical she could not make out my words. I called a few other people, including my co-worker, and she asked me what she should tell people - twins or triplets? I said, "Triplets. There are three babies in my belly!"

We went home for Christmas. It was a very long 3 hour drive for us. Our families were so confused and shocked. I visited with some friends, Matt and Michelle. They had to come see me because I could only sit against a pillow, my back hurt so badly. That night, had I known I would be in such pain, I would have gone to the E.R. I had no idea what was wrong, just that we were pregnant with triplets and one had passed away. Our family pastor laid hands on me and had the whole church pray over us. As I left the church that day, I remember the pastor, who has known me my whole life, saying, "Emily, this time next year, you will have three little babies on your lap!"

Did I mention that I was in denial, and I did not believe that Drake (Baby C) was dead? I would not believe that so-called doctor, anyway. I told people that we were having triplets, and I never told them that one had already died. Ronnie, Radd, and Hannah went from kissing my belly with one kiss to kissing it three times. It was great!

MARTIN: Next visit, we had another ultrasound and we thought the doctor was being funny when he told us our twins were fine. "What?!?!" is all we could say. We didn't have twins on either side of our family. "See this elongated body? Here's a head and here's feet.

Well, this head is for this heartbeat, and these feet are for this faint heartbeat," he said, and told us that he thought we were already informed about the twins. I didn't know what to feel. I was smiling, laughing, and crying all at once. I was so scared. I was unsure of my capability to handle two babies at once. I was so stunned; I didn't know what to say. We called our family and told everyone. I was still in disbelief until I saw two separate bodies on the next ultrasound. Those first few months, I couldn't keep ANYTHING down. I was as sick as a dog. My whole body went haywire. My moods were totally uncontrollable and I would argue with my husband for no reason, then the next minute be crying. I had such hatred toward everything. I didn't want to be touched or anything else. I was NOT myself by any means. I didn't like the person that I turned into.

<u>TUMMERS:</u> At 11 weeks and 2 days, I had my ultrasound and blood work done. I am a rather chatty person, and was telling the tech that I was so much smaller this time around and hadn't gained any weight at all. I couldn't get over how long this scan seemed to be taking. My husband hadn't shown up before I came in for the scan, so the tech said she'd go out and see if he was there now. She came back in and said he wasn't there, and that was too bad, because she had, she said, "some news for me …there's two babies in there". I teared up as she showed me the two babies for the first time, but not with tears of sadness or even of joy… just of disbelief at the amazing thing that was happening.

I was absolutely shocked and had no clue at all that I was carrying twins. I kept thinking, "How are we going to do this? How will we make this work?" My husband wasn't with me, but I quickly tried to find him once I got out of the office. When I finally found him he was wondering what I was so bent out of shape about. "What is it, twins?" he joked. I burst into tears and said yes. He was great about it, but then again, he had no clue what it takes to run a household financially. That's my role in our family. He was absolutely ecstatic.

I called my mom on the way to my hometown for a big rural festival of sorts, and told her to sit down. She asked why, and when I told her what I'd just found out, she just kept saying, "No way, no way," and laughing. By the time I saw her and my dad, about 2 hours later, half the town knew and everyone was so very excited. It was a catching feeling, and I soon became pretty excited myself.

LIGHT: We had an ultrasound earlier than usual because I had been having cramps and severe nausea. I remember being terrified of the worst, but never imagined it could be twins! So we were quite surprised to see two little peanuts on that screen.

CHRISTMAN-SCHARER: I had an appointment with my ob-gyn, Dr. G. I went to this appointment by myself because usually there is not much happening. I was 6 weeks, 4 days pregnant. Dr. G. did an internal ultrasound. He had the screen turned towards me, and I knew what to look for after going through it three previous times. I kept watching him scan back and forth, and I thought I saw two little spots on the screen, but I didn't think too much of it. Then my doctor turned the screen toward himself and said, "Uh-oh?!" I asked him, "What?" And with a smile on his face he said, "You are having twins!" Well, my reaction was not a happy one at first. I was scared, excited, and shocked. I was crying and saying that I couldn't have twins because I already had three boys at home. How was I going to do this? My doctor was concerned right away, saying he only saw one placenta and that he did not see a membrane separating them. He said the outcome would not be good, if that was the case. Well, of course, I was sitting there thinking, "Now that I am pregnant with these two babies, they will be ok and they will make it."

I must have sat with the nurse for quite a while. She gave me all the instructions for being pregnant with twins, and my prenatal vitamins. I had to take two of them at a time. Yuck! I was in a daze the whole time I was with her, wondering how I would take care of them and the three boys. Reid wasn't even a year old yet. My estimated due date was September 15, 2006; Reid would turn one on June 4. What was Karl going to say? He was totally shocked when I told him I was pregnant with Reid. He was 36 when I had Reid, his first child. I think at this point my doctor told me about twin to twin transfusion syndrome as well.

After I got out of the appointment, I went to my van, called Karl, and told him we were having twins. He was shell shocked, I think. I called my mom and told her I couldn't do it and she said I could. My dad was happy as well! He said, "Maybe these will be your girls!" The next day I went to St Luke's Hospital for genetic counseling. Because I was 37, they wanted to make sure everything was ok with the babies. After the testing, I went from having the statistics of a 37 year old, to those of a 21 year old. What a relief.

Let me tell you something. When I was pregnant with my first son, we didn't want to know what sex he was. They told my grandmother, who had Alzheimer's, and she said, "I know Shelley is pregnant and she is having a boy." Wow, what a surprise when that is what I had! When I was pregnant with the twins, someone told my grandfather, who has dementia, that I was having twins and he said, "I know, she is having two girls." Well, guess what, he was right! How weird is that?

MORGAN: It seems like yesterday when I had my first ultrasound. The ultrasound tech said, "Is this your first ultrasound?" My husband, who was sitting to my left, answered. She said, "Well…you have two babies in here. Was everyone saying that you'd have twins?" I called my mother and she said she wasn't surprised. Don't ask me why. Identical twins don't run in our family. I was shocked, but my husband almost fell out of his chair! He was also so excited. I will never forget that wonderful memory. We printed out pictures. We knew for sure one of the babies was a boy, not sure of the other. They couldn't tell at the time that they were identical. I was 14 weeks along. Right after my first ultrasound confirmed I was pregnant with twins, I began experiencing occasional severe lower backaches. I couldn't sleep lying down, so I had to sleep sitting upright on our couch. I thought the lower backaches were a normal, common sign of pregnancy.

REBILAS: It wasn't until my ultrasound at 20 1/2 weeks that we were told we were having twin boys and that we needed to go and see a perinatal doctor. We were on cloud nine. To look at the screen and see two little faces looking up at us was amazing! When they sent us to the perinatal doctor, we just assumed it was because it was twins; we had no idea what they were going to tell us next.

JELLEY: We decided we had better do an ultrasound right away. I had no idea when I was due since I hadn't had a period at all. So we scheduled one for that Thursday - 4 days away.

Thankfully, Cody called me as I was driving home that night. He said he was allowed a three minute phone call to let me know he had made it safely to the fort where he was training. I had to interrupt him, "I have to tell you something." He stopped talking, "I'm pregnant". He paused and said, "That's awesome baby; ok I have to go."

The night before the ultrasound I kept dreaming about the ultrasound. In my dream, I was told that I was having triplets and my due date was September 30th. I got up and wrote my husband a letter. I told him about the dream, and how I was already having those pregnancy dreams. I asked what he would think of having twins. It didn't even occur to me that I could have more naturally.

So my mom and I made it to the appointment, and Sherry, a midwife working with the doctor, began the ultrasound. As she started, the doctor asked how I knew I was pregnant. I told her there was a positive pregnancy test. As soon as we could see anything, the doctor said, "Whoa, let me take over." There was a series of "Do you see that?" and "I see that." My first thought was "Is there no baby? Maybe it was a false positive? She just asked if I was for sure pregnant." Finally, we asked, "WHAT?" And someone said, "It's twins." I asked (or yelled), "Are you serious?!" I had to be told that I couldn't sit up. After that, it's kind of like I was in a dream, looking at someone else's ultrasound. They found another baby and I was so numb I was just waiting for them to find more. Maybe this person in this dream was going to have a baby everywhere they looked. I seemed to get back to reality, looked at all the pictures, and finally got it in my head that there were three babies, not two, not five. Three. It became difficult for the doctor to answer questions, because we just kept coming up with more. My feelings were mixed. The thought of three babies was overwhelming. Plus, I like going to midwives, not doctors. I'd had two very good, easy births and now I was told I was going to have to have a c-section. At that point, I knew that the chance of multiples having special needs was higher, and that the chance of losing the babies was higher, too. I said right away, "My life is going to change, even if I can't keep these babies. I'll still be completely different."

In the next few weeks, I found that the odds of having spontaneous triplets, at my age, is about 1 in 10,000.

BENNER: My pregnancy was very normal. I didn't have morning sickness. I thought it was weird because I had heard about other women who had it horribly. I was just very tired all the time. I had always hoped that we would have twins. We knew it was a possibility, since I have an aunt and uncle that are twins.

At 10 weeks 5 days, we went for our first ultrasound. I was going to see a midwife. She started, and I didn't know what to expect to see on the screen. She paused and said, "Oh my god!" We replied, "What?!" I thought something was wrong and my heart stopped. "You guys are having twins." I started crying, Jacob was in shock, and we couldn't believe it had come true. At that point, the midwife told me that I was a high risk pregnancy and that she had to put me in the care of Dr. M. We just were so shocked and happy to be bringing two miracles into the world. From the beginning, we knew it was POSSIBLE that we could have twins. I had always dreamed of it, and hoped. My wish came true.

HOPE: The time for our 12 week ultrasound had finally come around. I was nervous and also very excited. Twins had never really come up, except with my father in law, who kept telling me, "You will have to buy two of everything." Then he would laugh and walk off.

My ultrasound started well, but within the first few moments the radiologists face changed. She got this really strange look and I started to panic, thinking there was something really wrong. She asked if I'd had really bad morning sickness. I said, "Yes, why are you asking?" She replied, "I'm not quite sure...I have never found twins before, but I'm pretty sure I see two babies." David and I looked at each other in shock, and then I just started laughing. My immediate thoughts were: there was no way I was having twins, no one I know has had twins, it would be impossible. David, on the other hand, was just so over the moon he couldn't wipe the smile from his face. A senior radiologist entered and continued the ultrasound. He confirmed that there were definitely two babies. He took all the measurements and had a good look around, but it was clear that something was not quite right. I asked if everything was ok, and he said, "I just need to check a few things." David leaned down and whispered, "I think there is something wrong with Twin B." The radiologist explained that he had picked up a significant size difference between the two babies, which we would need to discuss with our GP.

WRIGHT: When I was about seven weeks pregnant, I started cramping really badly. I was so scared that I was going to miscarry again. Crying, I headed to the emergency room, just sure that I was going to lose our baby. I was wheeled into ultrasound , but since I had come in through the ER, the tech wouldn't show me the monitor. I laid there and told her "our story." I told her that we were very excited about this pregnancy, that I am a fraternal twin, that my twin sister has identical twin girls, but that all of my other pregnancies were single births. After she finished scanning me, she leaned over and said, "I'm not supposed to tell you this, but not only did your sister have twins, you're having twins, too!" I couldn't believe it. She told me to act surprised when the ER docs told me. I was in a daze. My husband had joked about how cool it would be if we had twins, so when I called him overseas and told him, he thought I was joking.

DILLE: During my week 7 ultrasound, while the tech was scanning me, I wasn't watching the screen much, afraid I had miscarried when I spotted at 5 ½ weeks. Then, the ultrasound tech looked at me and asked if I could see what she saw. I looked at the screen and saw two babies. I said, "Um, there are two babies?" She said, "Yes, you are having twins!" I was in a complete state of shock, and told her that now I knew why I felt so strange. So many thoughts went through my head. What would my husband think? How could we afford twins, when we weren't even trying to get pregnant in the first place? What would my other kids think?

I had always wanted to have twin girls. It just seemed like it would be such fun to have two babies together, to see how they would interact, the relationship that they would have with one another. I was a bit scared about the timing, with two other children already at home. When we first found out that we were pregnant, some people told us we were going to have twins. I'm not sure why, and no one had ever said that about my two previous pregnancies. Though my husband's mother is a twin and I also have twin uncles, we just couldn't believe it actually happened to us.

BRAY: On the 28th of December, we were at my aunt's wedding. My grandfather was a twin, which almost everyone at the wedding brought to my attention, saying, "Wouldn't it be lovely if you had twins?", and "They say it skips a generation." I brushed it off and laughed. I didn't really believe that I would get pregnant with twins. December 29th came. Our appointment was late in the afternoon. The three of us waited for my name to be called. William was surprisingly well behaved, and sat on daddy's knee like a good boy. Our turn finally came. I laid on the bed and the nurse put the jelly on my tummy and began the scan. She looked at me and said, "I can see a pregnancy, but you need to go back out and drink more water. Your bladder is not full enough." After what felt like a very long 10 minutes, we went back and started again. By that point, William had started to get a little agitated. Gareth tried to settle him by saying, "Look at the little baby on the screen", to which the nurse replied, "Baby? Don't you mean babies? There's more than one in there." My heart stopped beating! "Twins!", I shouted, "Oh my God, we are having twins!" I looked at Gareth and he had the biggest smile on his face. "I thought I could see two," he said. I was in so much shock and was so happy. We honestly felt like the luckiest couple in the world, so special, to be given the gift of twins. Then the nurse explained that she needed to do an internal scan to get a better look. She stated that she needed to make sure both twins had their own amniotic sacs. It was after the scan that she said, "I'm not 100% sure but it looks as though your twins are identical. The good news is they both have their own amniotic sacs." She stated that it looked as if the twins were monochromic, diamniotic twins (each twin has its own sac but they share a placenta). Nothing else was said. We were taken to see the midwife then, who told us that as we were carrying twins, we would have to be consultant led. We were given an appointment for my 20 weeks gestation scan, and an appointment to see the midwife in a month's time. Nobody gave us any advice on twin pregnancy. Nobody told me that my pregnancy was now very high risk. Nobody mentioned TTTS.

OROSZ: They told us we were right, that there were two. We kind of already knew, since we'd had an "off the record" ultrasound, but it was confirmed by our OBGYN. Tears ran down my face; I was scared and happy all at the same time. We were shocked and surprised and excited, too. Everyone was very happy for us because twins run in my family. I never imagined I would have twins.

FLETCHER: I remember our first appointment with our doctor, on January 8th, 2008. I remember sitting in the waiting room, ready to be called back for our first ultrasound. Then the ultrasound tech, Pam, called us back for the ultrasound. I remember her looking at me and saying "How do you guys feel about two babies?" I remember crying, Scott looking about ready to pass out, and Austin saying, "I am going to have two sisters." I remember asking her to say what she had just said again. Then I looked up at the screen, and there they were - two little babies growing inside of me. I remember thinking, "Lord, I just prayed for one, but thank you for blessing me with two." This was a new ballgame for us. I remember finishing up the ultrasound and going to wait in another room to do the rest of the labs and all of that. I remember going in to see the doctor, who told us our twins were identical, no doubt. I thought,

"This is so cool!" I don't remember thinking about how we were going to do this. I was on cloud 9!

That was the first time we ever heard the words "Twin to twin transfusion syndrome". The doctor gave us all of the percentages about everything that can happen with a twin pregnancy. In your head, you think, "That will never happen to us." After leaving the doctor's office, we called everyone and told them it was twins. Some of their reactions were so funny to me, and I beamed from ear to ear. The looks on people's faces were priceless when we showed them the ultrasound pictures.

DOBBS: June 21, 2005, Dr. P. did another ultrasound and left the room. I looked at my husband as we waited for the news that it wasn't a viable pregnancy. Dr. P. returned with the ultrasound technician, who looked at Dr. P. and confirmed two. Dr. P. then turned to us and said, "You are having twins." My husband looked at me and said, "No we are not." I started to cry, yet was the happiest I had ever been.

I guess you could say that I was not one hundred percent shocked when we found out we were having twins, as this was the 13th set on my mother's side, and Michael's mother's twin died at birth, too small to survive. The larger twin was around 7 to 8 pounds, the smaller one around 3 pounds.

WALLINGTON: We went into the office at 8 weeks and were shocked to learn I was pregnant again, with twins. It scared me to death, as I worried I would have another miscarriage.

BRUCE: It was April 20, 2007, when we found out that I was carrying twins. I was 9 weeks, with a due date of November 25th. We were shocked! My husband more so than I; he turned ghost white and looked as if he was going to faint. Our ultrasound tech was so excited for us, though. After she announced I was carrying twins, she went on and on about us having to buy matching outfits, a twin stroller and just two of everything! I never once thought my mother-in-law's teasing would turn out to be true! After we got over the shock, and my mother-in-law stopped jumping up and down, screaming with joy, we felt special and somehow chosen that God would see fit to give us two precious gifts.

7
THE FIRST TRIMESTER THROUGH 13 WEEKS

BRUCH: I had regular OB appointments, but knew, in my heart, that something was wrong.

SLICHTER: The following two weeks, waiting for my next appointment, were torture for me. I was at the beginning of my 13th week, and after what felt like an eternity, I finally had the appointment with the high risk specialist. As he was doing the scan, he said he did not see a cystic hygroma, and I was so relieved. It felt like a huge weight was lifted off of my chest and I could finally breathe again. He said that the twins were most likely identical, due to a shared placenta and that he could see a very fine membrane separating the twins, therefore they each had their own sack. But he still had a very concerned look on his face. He excused himself and went back to his office. After a few minutes, he came back and said that one baby was smaller and had less amniotic fluid, which was not a good thing. He informed us that most likely I had Twin-to-Twin Transfusion Syndrome. I had no idea what that was, so my husband and I flooded him with questions, and were not happy about the answers we received. He explained to us exactly what it was, why it was happening and how we could treat it. He went on to say that having this condition early on in a pregnancy was not something he considered a good thing, and there that was a significant chance that we would lose both twins. Though he was a pro-life doctor, he told us our first option was to terminate. My husband and I did not like the idea of that, so we refused and said we would let nature take its course.

MARTIN: On Fathers' Day, I started bleeding. Just a little bit. I had been so excited to make it past the miscarriage mark, like the books said. But the next day it was like a GUSH! Like something filled with blood had opened and closed, so I FREAK OUT and we rush to the ER. To my surprise, this new hospital was on their toes. The first doctor told me that my placenta was ripping from the wall. They sent me home. I followed up with my OB, who told me it was a clot. I was confused and I just prayed that my OB was right. He told me that the clot would be absorbed, provided it never got any bigger. After about a week or two, the clot was nowhere to be seen on my ultrasounds, though I was still spotting.

DICK: I found out I was pregnant early in my first trimester. I just figured I had to be pregnant. I didn't feel like I was sick with a cold but I kept throwing up. I craved ice cream non-stop and had to take naps constantly. I felt drained, but I was extremely happy to be so drained, because I knew I had created life and it was growing inside of me.

TUMMERS: My brother was getting married in mid-October and expecting their first baby about 3 weeks before my due date. I got a dress altered for that wedding, made smaller actually, in mid-August. When I went for my final dress fitting my mom and I were shocked to discover that I needed the dress let back out in my upper abdominal area. It was then, at 13 weeks, that we realized how much I was showing already. I couldn't get over how tired I felt at night and yet how energized I was during the day. I was very active for someone as overweight as I was; I had actually been working at losing weight with the help of a dietician before getting pregnant. I had lost 25 pounds and was eating so well.

In week 13, I had a follow up appointment with my midwife. It was there we learned that our babes were identical. I had mistakenly thought, when the tech told me they each had their own sac, that it meant they were fraternal. I also learned then that I had an anterior placenta.

The midwife was unable to find the heartbeats, but wasn't too concerned since it was pretty early. She decided to send me for another ultrasound, mostly so that my husband could see the babies. It was done the next day and all went well, except this tech couldn't find the dividing membrane, and was very concerned. I was booked for another scan the following week. I began researching mono mono twins and mono di twins, and of course began to panic. Little did I know that learning they weren't mono mono did not put us out of the woods.

CHRISTMAN-SCHARER: We looked up all the information we could online so we would be prepared for this. I mean twins, TTTS -- it was just so much to take in all at once. I found a lot of information on the twin to twin transfusion syndrome foundation website. We told the boys I was pregnant with twins. They were excited. After I had Reid, they asked if we could have more babies.

My next appointment was at 8 weeks and 6 days. That was Thursday; we heard both heartbeats and they were both very strong. They sounded really good. The doctor put me on iron pills that day.

On Monday, at 12 weeks and 4 days, I had an ultrasound with Dr. S. at the local hospital perinatology center. We saw the twins. It was just so amazing to see the two of them there. The technician took an educated guess and said that they were girls but not to tell anyone yet. They would be able to confirm it at my next appointment. I was excited that they were girls. I was finally getting my girls. Not that I don't love my boys, but I really wanted a little girl and now I was blessed with identical twin girls!

I had another appointment, with my OB, on Monday and everything was ok. The heartbeats were strong. I was 13 weeks, 3 days at that point.

JELLEY: I had to wait until Sunday to tell my husband, because he wasn't able to call sooner. He did the same thing I did, in shock, there was no reaction. I told him and I think he just paused and went on with his thought from before I told him. But both of us were extremely excited that we were having triplets, which is not something that happens every day.

My next ultrasound was three weeks later, at 10 weeks, and the doctor mentioned TTTS. She was saying that some desperate parents do some laser thing even though it doesn't do anything; really there is nothing you can do. I don't know when it was that I asked her to explain what TTTS was, but she said it was a blood flow issue.

My next appointment was made with the perinatologists in Missoula, 3 and ½ hours away. I was 12 weeks. He was very professional, but seemed a little short when we asked too many questions. After he was all done scanning, he began to tell me something was wrong. I remember thinking that for having to tell someone something that awful, he had sure done it in a nice but professional way, not overly caring nor too cold. Baby A had hydrops, which was fluid under the skin. It was everywhere; I remember wishing that he would stop showing me more places with fluid. He said it could be TTTS, an anatomy problem (e.g. heart defect), or a chromosome problem. He pointed out that there was only one placenta, which meant that the babies were identical, so if it was chromosomal, they would all have it. He sent me away after saying that most likely I would end up with a normal twin pregnancy, that at the next appointment; baby A would most likely be gone. He said I would have no signs of miscarriage; the baby would be a disappearing twin and just flatten out on the side. I went away very numb and wanting my husband. I couldn't cry, couldn't talk, and couldn't move. I asked everyone with me not to tell anyone, because I just wasn't ready. I texted Cody to tell him I needed to talk, so when he called that night, he knew something wasn't right. I honestly don't remember our conversation, I just remember the next few days, when he could call (he had to sneak every call since they weren't supposed to have phones), he would reassure me that everything was going to be ok and that God was going to take care of us and baby A. I found that without my husband, I couldn't cry. I was irritable but not emotional. But in those next 3 weeks I prayed a lot. I was finally able to tell people and asked everyone to pray for Gods Will, and for him to help us though whatever that was.

We found out that the odds of having identical

triplets are actually somewhat unknown. I saw 1 in 1 million a lot, with the argument that it could be as much as 500 million. Because TTTS is only in 10% of twins, it doesn't happen much, either. When someone said, "Don't worry about getting that, that's rare," I learned to say, "Really? Look at my identical triplets, hello? Who cares how rare it is, I'll get it."

HOPE: Walking into the OB's office I was very nervous. So many thoughts had been running through my head, and David's intuition had been telling him it wasn't going to be a good day. The receptionist informed me that she had been trying to contact me; since the OB I was seeing didn't deliver twins, they were unable to help us. I understood, but asked that since we were there, would the doctor discuss the ultrasound results with us. The OB called us in and apologized for having to deliver such bad news. It was her opinion, due to the results, that Twin B was suffering from Down syndrome or the like. She felt we needed to start discussing our options. At this stage, there was 2 weeks and 3 days growth difference between them. She gave us a referral to a specialist OB in a town 2 hours away. We were both devastated. It was hours before we could speak to each other, and then all we could do was cry. My mum drove down that night to be with us for a week. I was barely coping and all I could say or think was, "I am not going to lose one of my babies!"

- I must note at the time, we lived in a town called Griffith, in NSW, Australia. It is toward the middle of NSW, and has a population of 15,000 people. The nearest major city was 2 hours away. Medical resources were very limited.

WRIGHT: At 13 weeks, I had my first visit with the perinatologists. I found out that week that we were expecting identical twin girls! During the ultrasound, the technician brought in her supervisor and one of the doctors. They each took turns scanning my babies. I had no idea what was going on. The next thing I knew, I was in a room with one of the perinatologists from the high-risk group, and a medical student. This was the first time I ever heard the words "Twin to twin transfusion syndrome". I was devastated. I was told that Sarah (Baby A) was 30% smaller than her sister Julie Anne (Baby B). I was told that I needed to do Selective Reduction and "cut the cord" to Sarah, or that I needed to terminate the pregnancy and "start over". I replied flat out that I was not going to kill either of my babies, and that whatever I could do to save both of my girls, I was going to do. I was told that Sarah would probably die and then Julie Anne would die, too, and that I needed to just end it now. I went home and Googled everything I could about TTTS. My husband even started researching thousands of miles away, overseas.

DILLE: I was at almost 13 weeks when I got the flu. I ended up in the ER because I couldn't eat or drink anything and I was worried about the babies. I received IV fluids and was monitored for a few hours. The doctors also sent me for an ultrasound to check on the babies. I couldn't believe how much they had grown since our last ultrasound. They were starting to look like little people! The ultrasound tech and doctor told me that they both looked great; they had great heartbeats and were very active.

BRAY: I was at the start of my second trimester and working full time. Everybody kept commenting on how big I was. I laughed it off and thought nothing of it. I was carrying twins, so I was going to be larger than average. There were two little babies growing inside me after all. At the end of January 2009, I was due to see the midwife. The appointment went well; I got to hear both babies' heartbeats and the midwife seemed happy. So I was happy.

OROSZ: The first trimester I was very sick with morning sickness. I couldn't keep anything down. It was confirmed at 7 weeks that I was carrying twins. I wouldn't say that my morning sickness was any worse than with my first son. I didn't throw up as much, but I craved fruits and tomato juice a lot.

FLETCHER: The first trimester went by pretty well, besides the ALL Day morning sickness. I had never been so sick before in my life. I knew this pregnancy was different for sure. Doctor's visits went well and the labs were all good. Everything was looking great, until I hit 13 weeks and started bleeding that Friday. I was put on bed rest for a few days to see if it would stop. It did, for a little while. On Monday, when I went back to see the doctor, they put me back on bed rest. This would seem like the longest bed rest ever.

DOBBS: The pregnancy moved right along. On July 19, 2005, I just happened to be seeing Dr. P. again and he said that everything looked fine. He agreed that I needed to see him every two weeks. The next month was pretty uneventful.

BRUCE: The first trimester went by quickly. We found out that we were expecting twins at 9 weeks gestation and we continued with regular doctor appointments. My belly grew at rapid speed and the idea of having twins settled with our family and friends. The pregnancy was being nice to me and I experienced no morning sickness or nausea. I just kept getting bigger and I was extremely content with that.

8
Week 14

SLICHTER: The doctor wanted me to begin weekly ultrasounds. In my 14th week, there were small signs of improvement. The donor showed some signs of increased amniotic fluid, which was an absolutely good thing. The doctor said he hadn't grown much, but there was an improvement from the preceding week. As for the recipient, his fetal measurements were consistent with his gestational age; he was growing well and was doing wonderfully. I then saw some hope, and felt things would take a turn for the better.

TUMMERS: The ultrasound tech was fantastic, though confusing. She was able to find the membrane, and surprised when I commented that this made them identical. She questioned why I was sure, as this wasn't known for certain yet. I still have no idea why she said that mono-di meant identical. But ironically enough, my doctor also made comments to that effect. I wonder now if something looked odd to them, made them think there was something there.

WRIGHT: After going home and reading everything I could on TTTS, I talked to my doctor and asked him about starting protein shakes and bed rest. He said to try it if I wanted, and we would see if it helped. I started drinking protein shakes immediately, but since I was still working full-time, I could only rest before and after work.

DILLE: I had a routine OB checkup that week. I got to hear the babies' heartbeats with the Doppler and also had a quick ultrasound to check on the babies' growth. Dr. B. told me that both babies looked great and still had strong heartbeats.

OROSZ: Had another ultrasound at 14 weeks because I was having horrible pains in my back and sides. Nothing was found to be wrong. I remember asking the ultrasound tech about TTTS, and she told me she thought I was "past the stage to get it at 14 weeks." She had no idea what Twin to Twin was.

FLETCHER: The bleeding seemed to have slowed down a lot. The fear of losing my babies was the feeling in the world. I felt so helpless, but other than the bleeding and the all-day morning sickness, everything was looking normal.

9
Week 15

SLICHTER: The next appointment went well. Although there wasn't much improvement, things hadn't gotten any worse. We were very happy about that, although we wished things were improving a little bit faster.

MARTIN: After about two months, the bleeding stopped. But another problem arose. I had gained a lot of weight, between 7 and 9 pounds a month. My ankles were swelling already. I looked like I was 7 months along. My doctor constantly told me that I was FAT and needed to stop eating anything white: bread, potatoes, even milk. Every time I went into the office – at least every week or so -- he put me down. I DREADED going. I truly wasn't eating all that much. My ankles were "kankles"; I had stretch marks on my legs and arms. I was HUGE!

JELLEY: I was doing ok. Then, the night before my next appointment, my husband's cousin (who was pregnant and due the same time as I) called to say she had lost the baby. It had been twins, and from what they could gather, she had miscarried one the week before. It must have messed with her enough that she couldn't carry the other one. We found out later that her doctor's best guess was TTTS.

I went to my next appointment praying for the same or better news. The first thing I asked was if there were still three heartbeats. I could see movement everywhere and it really looked like 3 babies. This time we had an ultrasound tech; she was really patient and answered any questions that she could.

So she showed me baby A's heartbeat before she did her little routine. I thanked God and waited for the doctor to come tell me about baby A. When he came, he said baby A no longer had hydrops. There was no fluid under the skin, and from what he could see, everybody looked good. We were too excited to really listen to what he said after that. He mentioned that baby A had more fluid than babies B and C, which could be a sign of TTTS. He went on to explain if it was TTTS, I would go to WA or UT and have the connections lasered. I honestly didn't know why he was even talking about that when everything was fine.
All of my babies were the same size and looked great. I wasn't worried. I thought whatever was wrong had corrected itself, and that all the doctor was doing was telling me what could happen.

BENNER: On my second ultrasound at 15 weeks, Dr. M. mentioned TTTS. It crossed my mind and I should have researched it more, but I didn't. I think I was still shocked to be caring for TWO babies. He did verify that there was a separating membrane and everything was normal.

HOPE: We arrived at the specialist very sedate and quiet. He read all the results, performed another ultrasound, and stated that the other one was wrong and there was a size difference of only three days. He sent us away with an appointment for a follow up ultrasound, in two weeks' time, back in our own town. By this time, though, the damage was already done. We knew things weren't right, and although they didn't appear to be as bad as first thought, it was very hard to shake what we had already been through. I found it very hard to enjoy my pregnancy.

I must note, it was at this stage that I found out our town had a twins club. I rang Melissa, its President, and burst into tears explaining what had gone on. She was lovely, and invited me to a twins' picnic that weekend. The parents at that picnic welcomed us with open arms. They talked about the bumps in the road and offered support. They became some of the most precious people in our lives over the next few months. Not a week went by without a call from one of them or a visit. It was comforting, and I began to learn a lot about what it was going to be like to be a mother of twins.

WRIGHT: My 15 week ultrasound showed a little bit of improvement in the disparity between my girls. Sarah was now only 27% smaller than her sister, and she had a bit more fluid around her. The doctor felt that if the bed rest and the protein shakes had helped in just one week, we could try this avenue to help my girls. I was immediately put on bed rest, allowed only to take care of my other children. I concentrated on the protein shakes and eating healthy for my girls.

FLETCHER: I remember that week like it was yesterday. I remember having an ultrasound and finding out it was GIRLS! Allyson Jean and Abbigail Laken.: "Allybug" and "Abbygal". The ultrasound was going well; Pam was looking at the membrane that separated them. She called in Dr. B., my OB/GYN, and he looked also. That is when we heard the words we dreaded, twin to twin transfusion syndrome. It is amazing how you can go from cloud nine to such fear and helplessness, all in a few minutes. After the ultrasound, I talked to Dr. B. He told us everything we needed to know. I was scheduled to see a high risk doctor. Our lives changed in a moment. The fight of our daughters' lives, and ours, had begun. Our faith would be put to the test.

10
Week 16

BRUCH: This ultrasound went fine, no major issues; they didn't say anything was wrong. I found out why I wasn't feeling my babies move, though. My placenta was located on my belly, so it was acting like a cushion, or barrier, between us. I really wanted to feel them, even if I would be kept up late at night from the movement. Then, I found out that we were to have boys and that they were fine. Their names would be Vincent Sterling and Thomas Matthew. "Sterling" was the namesake of my husband's grandfather. "Thomas" was my father, and grandfather, and great grandfathers, and great-great grandfather. "Matthew" came from my brother, and also my brother- in-law.

HADDIGAN: They sent us to a specialist for our 16 week appointment to verify size, check for identicals, and make sure that there was a separating membrane. The specialist looked at the babies and told us we were having boys! My 7 year old son was thrilled - he couldn't imagine having two sisters! Then, the tech said she was concerned about fluid levels and was going to have the doctor come in to look. The doctor verified what she saw. There was a considerable difference in fluid levels. We would need to come back in two weeks to have things measured.

SLICHTER: At the 16th week ultrasound, measurements were similar to week 15. No major improvements, but then again, no signs of recession on either twin. The donor was still quite small, and still had little amniotic fluid. The recipient was growing perfectly and doing fine, showing no signs of normal recipient symptoms. His heart was doing well and had a normal steady beat.

DICK: After the ultrasound appointment, the head tech said he wanted to send me to a high-risk specialist because I was only 18 and having identical twins for my first pregnancy. I didn't think anything about seeing a specialist; I figured the doctors knew what they were doing. I was scheduled to meet with the specialist at the very end of May, 2007. I couldn't wait to hear what they had to say. I knew they were going to take good care of me.

TUMMERS: I began seeing the OB that had delivered both my boys during week 16. We had some good laughs when he asked if I'd been taking anything to get pregnant. I asked him about drinking protein drinks, as I had read about that in a few books. He was adamant that I not drink them, and told me that the best nutritional plan was the gestational diabetic diet. It is pretty similar to what I had followed to lose weight: lots of protein- rich foods combined with whole grains, veggies and fruit.

We talked about when I'd be ordered off work (28 weeks), and discussed the reasons for this (including preterm labor). He admitted he had no real concerns about that, given my history; I don't go into labor on my own - both of our sons were born 10 or more days overdue. Instead, he told me that his biggest concern was growth, and more specifically, any difference in growth between the two babies. I asked him if he was talking about TTTS, and he said he was, as well as about other growth issues in identical twins.

He also scared me, giving me a list of restrictions a mile long. He wrote me a letter for work, to ensure that I was not on my feet for any length of time, or doing anything remotely physical, including yard duty (I work as an Educational Assistant). The wording in this letter was "very high risk pregnancy - patient to be off her feet as much as possible". That led to a lot of stress at work, since my boss was very bizarre about how he dealt with this news. Over-compensation would be putting it mildly. It was odd to be treated with such kid gloves, and hard to accept that I was going to have to slow down and be careful. My scans were booked for just before 18 weeks and then 5 weeks after that.

CHRISTMAN-SCHARER: I had another appointment with the perinatologists and Dr. B. Everything was looking ok. My fluid and cervix were good and they said they were 99% sure the babies were girls. My mom, Tyler and Alex had come to this appointment, and we were all very excited that I was having girls. Now, don't get me wrong, I love my boys, but I always wanted a girl. What a gift! I was getting two girls exactly alike. What more could you ask for?

I continually got getting bigger and bigger. My belly was bigger than when I was pregnant with my boys, but I thought it was just because I was having twins.

BENNER: At 19 weeks, on December 13, my Mom, Jacob and I went to the hospital to find out the sex. I had been hurting in my side, but I thought it was just my abdomen stretching, of course, carrying two babies! Baby A was definitely a boy and he was proud of it, but we weren't so sure about Baby B. The ultrasound techs spent half an hour looking and had me turn every which way. I didn't know what was going on, but they were looking for the separating membrane, as it was hard to find now. When we went to see Dr. M, he said, "They were a little concerned about the ultrasound." He looked for himself, and said, "I'm sending you to OKC, to OU medical center, to see a specialist." My heart stopped when he said, "I think you may have TTTS." He told us, briefly, that the babies had a small chance of surviving, but the numbers were very low. He made the appointment at OU for the following week. I told him about the pain I was having, and he just told me to stretch and use a heating pad. We left the hospital numb and confused.

When we got to the parking lot, my phone rang. It was the doctor. OU wanted to see me ASAP and I should expect a phone call from them. Not even a mile away, my phone rang again and I had an appointment at OU the next day.

On December 14th, Jacob and I went to Oklahoma City to the OU Physicians of Maternal Fetal Medicine. The ultrasound tech was really great, and confirmed they were both boys! Dr. R came in and said, "You have Twin to twin transfusion syndrome and Two IDENTICAL BOYS." My heart stopped. He began to tell us everything about this horrible disease. I was in stage two of TTTS, with 15 cm of fluid in baby A's sac (average is 7-8cm). Because it was found before 24 weeks, I had severe TTTS.

Dr. R wanted to start an amnioreduction right then, since it would increase the probability of saving them. I had a 3and1/2 inch needle stuck through my abdomen, into my uterus, and into baby A's (Mason's) amniotic sac. Two liters were drained out. The pain in my side was relieved; I came to find out the TTTS was causing it. Over the next 4 weeks, I had weekly visits and a total of three amnioreductions. The babies would get better and get worse. The laser surgery was mentioned a few times, but we had hope that the amnio was going to work and so did my doctor.

HOPE: We had our next ultrasound and went off to our new OB to discuss the whole thing. This gentleman, Dr. C, was to become like family. He discussed the original results and determined that there was no evidence to support the theory of Down syndrome. In fact, he was amazed that we had been put through all that. Our latest ultrasound showed the growth difference back at 2 weeks 4 days. Though he did not see the need to panic, he wanted us to return for another ultrasound in two weeks. He gave us his home number and advised that if, at any time, we had even the slightest problem, we should contact him immediately. At this stage I was becoming very frightened. I hated talking about being pregnant. I cried most days, sitting and praying for the safety of my babies.

WRIGHT: The bed rest and the protein shakes seemed to be helping! The disparity had dropped to 22% and we were keeping the fluid levels within the acceptable range. My doctors had been talking about sending me for surgery to laser the connections between the babies, but we were told that the fluid levels had to be less than 2dvp and greater than 8dvp. Sarah's fluid level was right around 2.6dvp, and Julie Anne's was around 6.5dvp.

OROSZ: During week 16, I switched to a high risk

doctor. My original doctor's office was only open on Mondays, and couldn't give me the answers I wanted. I wasn't even told if they were identical or not. Her words were, "You will just have to wait until they are born and a few months old to see if they look alike or not." Now granted, I wouldn't have found out at 7 weeks that I was carrying twins if it weren't for my friend, but since we knew, I felt that I should already have had more ultrasounds. I feared if I stayed with her, neither of my twins would survive. After switching, the high risk doctor found they were identical BOYS. Then the doctor told us about TTTS, and what to look for. We decided to name the boys Blake and Carter.

FLETCHER: We were scheduled to see the high risk doctor. Dr. L was a wonderful and caring doctor. I remember the first time I met him, and the tech that did our ultrasounds. Her name was Erin and she was a sweet girl. They did the ultrasound to look at the girls and their TTTS. He talked about all of the things that could go wrong, and all of the things that could be done. I never heard the word "abortion" so many times in my life, but I know they have to talk about everything with you. We spoke about the two closest TTTS specialists. There was one in Pennsylvania, and one in Florida. Dr. L had worked with the one in Florida, so we felt more comfortable seeing him. Everything was set in motion, and we were on our way to see Dr. Q Hopefully, he could perform the surgery that might save both of our girls. At this point, all we could do was hope and pray. We knew God had his arms wrapped around our girls.

WALLINGTON: When we got to 16 weeks, we went to see the high-risk doctor in Tampa, Florida. That's when we found out that our little girls were suffering from Twin to Twin syndrome. The fear I had for my children was indescribable. I was sent to St. Joseph's hospital in Tampa, where I met Dr. Q. and Dr. C. These men are incredible and very compassionate doctors. First, I was told that the fluids were not at the right levels to be eligible for laser surgery, which might correct the uneven blood flow between my daughters. Then, Dr. C. did an ultrasound himself, and found, indeed, I was eligible. I was scheduled for surgery the next day. I could not understand why all this was happening to my children and me. I was terrified, and prayed and prayed for God to help them. I knew I had to be strong for what I was going to endure through the rest of my pregnancy. I knew I had to have Faith that the Lord would help us through this.

The surgery went well and I was sent home the next day, on bed rest. I was 16 weeks along, which is the earliest you can have the surgery. I continued seeing Dr. C. every week, to make sure that the girls were doing okay. Soon, we found out my donor baby, Lilly, was not growing as she should and was struggling. Lilly had Inter Uterine Growth Restriction and Dr. C. was unsure of her future.

Every week in his office, I would lie on the table trembling in fear, anticipating hearing her heartbeat. Every week, I thanked God for carrying us through these times. I kept my Faith strong; it was all I had.

11
Week 17

SLICHTER: At the 17th week ultrasound, I found out that our twins were BOYS! We were so happy and excited. We named them Jack (the donor) and Jake (the recipient). Jake was in perfect health, size, and amniotic fluid; there was nothing at all wrong with him. Jack wasn't doing as well as we all had hoped, and the doctor gave me the option to see a TTTS specialist at UNC. We happily agreed. I felt very lucky to be in North Carolina, because there was a brilliant TTTS specialist only two hours away at UNC Chapel Hill, which is a wonderful hospital.

CADLE: In week 17, I had gained 17 pounds, my B.P. was 142/78, and I was measuring 27 weeks. I could hardly breathe or walk! I was miserable. The doctor said nothing about Drake (baby C) being dead, just that he could not see me anymore. I would need to see a specialist. They would fax the referral, but I was told not to call, as they did not like it when patients called. So I went home and waited.

TUMMERS: My midwife measured me this time and I was measuring like I was 20 weeks…not too bad yet. I hadn't gained any weight at all and my vitals were great. We could faintly hear one heart beat and weren't worried at all.

CHRISTMAN-SCHARER: I had an appointment with my OB. Everything was ok. Heartbeats were good. I also had an appointment with the perinatologists. We were told that they thought TTTS had started. It was "wait and see"; I had to go back to get the fluid levels checked. They also talked about CHOP – Children's Hospital of Philadelphia—as it was very early in the pregnancy for this to start and they were very concerned. We named the girls Karlyn Nicole - Baby A and Kylie Marie - Baby B. I was feeling movement from them now.

JELLEY: I went to Missouri for Cody's graduation from basic training; I brought Eliza with me and left Gareth with my little sister. When I saw my husband, I could feel all of my emotions coming back, the ones I was too strong to allow. We got to the car and I just burst into tears. Even though I thought our babies were fine, the emotions still came back. I had been told my baby was going to die. I needed to cry about it and have him hold me. After a very emotional few days, I had to say goodbye again and go home. Cody went on to AIT for schooling, part of his training.

WRIGHT: My doctors contacted the surgery center in Cincinnati, Ohio. As I have family close to there, it would be easier for us to go if I were to have the laser ablation surgery. My doctor said that as soon as the fluid levels shifted, we would be on our way. Today's ultrasound showed both of my girls, happily kicking away. Everything had remained stable.

FLETCHER: I remember the day we left for Tampa. Two of our good friends, Jon and Sarah Thorp, went with us. We left thinking about how we were going to pay for this trip, but God already knew! We had so many people raising money for us; it was a blessing to know that so many people cared so much. A little over a thousand dollars was raised. Cheryl, a flight attendant who was a member at the credit union where I worked, even offered us her points to fly

Tampa. I had never been on a plane, though, and that scared me a little bit. It seemed like it would take forever to get to Tampa. I had started hurting losing fluid that week, so I was in pain all the way. We ran into a storm around Savannah, Georgia, and had to find a hotel room. It was tough to find one with the power still on, but we finally did. I think we slept for maybe two hours, then it was time to hit the road again.

We finally got to Tampa, checked into our hotel room, and tried to get some rest before going to Tampa General Hospital to see Dr. Q. Monday, March 17th, 2008, our lives would change again. I remember getting up early and heading to the hospital. I was still in unbearable pain, but I wouldn't tell anyone as I didn't want people to think I was whining. We got to the hospital, checked in and waited for what seemed like forever. The whole time, we were praying, praying and praying that we had made the right decision for Ally and Abby, that this surgery would work, and that God would take care of us all. Then it was time to go in and get our first ultrasound of the day. The tech's name was Rhonda and she was a very sweet lady. Scott and I asked her a thousand questions. After Rhonda was done, we had to wait on Dr. Q. I remember pain and feeling like I needed to use the bathroom. I knew this was a sign of labor and that put me into a panic, but I hid all of my concerns to try and stay strong for Scott. Then it was time to see Dr. Q. I knew from the moment I met him he would do whatever it took to help us. He did another ultrasound and talked about the surgery. Then, the room got silent for a few moments, and he turned to us with tears in his eyes. He said there was nothing we could do. "The membrane that separates the babies has come unattached from your uterine wall. If I do the surgery, there is a chance of you and the babies dying," he said. He told us that Ally had a knot in her cord, at her belly button. He felt so badly because we drove so far and there was nothing he could do to help us. I remember him saying, "I know people don't like hearing these words, and I don't like having to talk about it, but one option is abortion." I looked at him and said, "If anyone is going to take my babies from me, it will be God!" He totally understood where I was coming from. We couldn't live with the "What Ifs?" Dr. Q. told us to hope and to do a lot of praying.

Rhonda gave us some tissues and told us to take our time. We were both breaking down at that point. I thought it was over, but God had other things in store for us. I remember Scott asking "Why?" What had we done that had been so wrong to have to go through this? I told him that everything was going to be ok and God was going to take care of us - ALL OF US! We left and found Sarah and Jon. I didn't want to talk to anyone, but just broke down in the car, praying, "Lord, don't take my babies from me, PLEASE!" We went back to the hotel to call our family and friends and let them know that they couldn't do the surgery. Scott and I grew so much closer through this. We learned to lean on each other for support.

We left the next day to head back home, but made a detour to Clearwater to see the beach. We had promised Austin we would get him some seashells from Florida. I couldn't wait to see our little man Austin. A child's smile and hug can make you feel so much better, no matter what you are going through.

The day after we got home from Tampa, Dr. B. called to see how things had gone in Florida. I had to tell him the news. From that moment on, I knew that Dr. B. was an amazing doctor. He truly cared about us, and Ally and Abby. I knew we were in good hands.

BRUCE: On June 21, 2007, we went for our second ultrasound, at 17 weeks and 4 days gestation, with a Maternal Fetal Medicine doctor. My OB wanted me to see a Maternal Fetal Medicine doctor just because I was having twins. The ultrasound brought devastating news. Our twins were diagnosed with Twin-to-Twin Transfusion Syndrome. The doctor explained to us that it was a problem with the placenta, and that unless I was somehow able to grow a new placenta, the chances of my twins surviving were grim. He went on to tell us Baby A's chances were even more grim than Baby B's, because the ultrasound showed Baby A had hydrocephalus. We didn't know how to react. My mother and mother-in-law were present, and began to ask questions, but the doctor was ugly with them and told them he would only answer the questions of those covered under our insurance. He then told me that I was to begin bed rest immediately, lying on my left side for 23.5 hours a day. I was only allowed to get out of bed to shower and use the restroom. By putting me on bed rest, he hoped to even out the fluids in the twins' sacs by my next appointment. Looking back, I realize how uneducated my doctor was, because no amount of bed rest cures TTTS. As we left, my mother-in-law asked the ultrasound tech if the sex had been discovered, and the tech replied that we were having identical girls. We were heartbroken, and given not a single ounce of hope. I went home and began my bed rest, afraid that at any moment my girls would die. We named Baby A, Jordyn Lee, and Baby B, Taylor Lauren.

12
Week 18

BRUCH: After the ultrasound, the doctor came in and said our boys had TTTS. My world just shattered. I was so scared since I didn't know what it was. My husband wasn't with me; he had to work that day. How could I tell him we had a problem? I wanted my babies to be healthy, to be safe. I wondered what was happening, and why? How can they be saved? Could they really lead a normal life? I kept wondering if I would be able to hold them, watch them grow, kiss their booboos away. I wondered if I would even know the simplest parental joy, hearing their first cries. I knew I had to deal with this some way. I was put on bed rest for the remainder of the pregnancy, referred to CHOP, pulled from work, and told to wait by the phone for CHOP to call. I felt so helpless.

HADDIGAN: We spent two weeks reading everything we could on TTTS. I found that I should be lying on my left side and drinking all the high protein shakes I could handle. I did just that. We had no idea what we were in for at our next appointment. The doctor looked over everything. We thought the babies were moving better than they had been, so we were feeling relieved. The doctor explained that our babies were in trouble, and that if something wasn't done immediately, we would lose them both. Our donor had 2mm of fluid and our recipient had 16mm (normal is around 8). We needed to go home and pack to leave for Maryland Medical Center in the morning. We had no idea things would be moving in this direction, or this fast. We had to find a sitter for our 7 year old and book a hotel for the next few nights in Maryland.

The staff and doctor in Maryland were wonderful. They explained everything as they measured our little guys and told us they were perfect for the surgery. The recipient was having heart issues, and the donor was stuck and his bladder was not seen, but things were not so bad that it couldn't turn around. We spent that night in a hotel room, worrying about the next day and the risks we were taking. We had no choice if our boys were going to have a chance.

SLICHTER: During my 18th week, we went to UNC to meet with the TTTS specialist. He did an amniocentesis due to a suspected a cystic hygroma, as well as to test for any other chromosomal abnormalities. The test came back good, and there were no abnormalities. He did many other tests, that was when we found out that Jack also had a velamentous cord, a very rare condition where the umbilical cord isn't correctly attached to the placental mass, inserting instead on the chorion-amniotic membranes. The incidence of this condition in twin gestation is about 8.7%, and found more often in Monochorionic placentation, or when the placentas are fused, than when the placentas are non-fused. (The incidence of velamentous insertion is greater during early pregnancy; it has been estimated, in spontaneous abortions, to be 33% between weeks 9 and 12, and 26% between weeks 13 and 16.)

The specialist advised us that Jack had about 20% chance of surviving. He mentioned that he was very surprised that Jack had made it this long. He added that due to the sharing of blood, if Jack died in utero, it would cause Jake to become brain dead. Our options then became very limited.

CADLE: I waited and waited continuing to grow bigger. It was getting harder to walk and breathe. I remember going to the E.R. because I could not breathe and I had these tiny red dots all over my chest. I called my doctor, who said that he could not see me anymore, that I had to wait to hear from the specialist, but that if I thought I needed to be seen, I should go to the E.R. The weird thing is, they could not find a heartbeat, but they were using an old time Doppler and acted like they did not really care, anyway. So I went home and waited to hear from the specialist.

TUMMERS: My 18 week scan was done a bit too early for Baby B. He was too small to get all organs checked, so I was rescheduled for 13 days later. With each scan, I hoped to learn what sex my babes were, but they just didn't want to co-operate. I did get great pictures. It was so very cool to me to have those pictures and show them off.

CHRISTMAN-SCHARER: I went to the perinatologists. Dr. S. said that the girls looked good, but that they were on the verge of first stage TTTS; they would wait and see. We did all of our research on this, knew what we needed to know, and were very proactive with the doctors. My brother and his wife, who live in California, sent us identical outfits for the girls. Dr. S. kept telling us that we were more proactive and informed about TTTS than most parents.

A few days later, I had another appointment with the perinatologists. Things were the same. Nothing had changed, which was a good sign. If it stayed at the early stage as long as possible, it meant the best possible outcome for BOTH of our girls.

MORGAN: During a routine ultrasound, the doctor at Phoenix Perinatal saw minor differences in the amniotic fluid levels of the babies. He said that often the amniotic fluid goes back to normal, but scheduled an appointment for the following week.

JELLEY: I was getting really achy, but I had never been pregnant with triplets, so I just figured that was normal. I was starting to need to lay down all the time and moving became very difficult. The day before my 18 week appointment, I was worried, since I noticed that all the movement I was feeling had stopped in one spot. I went to the birth center and asked if Julia, my moms' assistant, could try and find heartbeats with the Doppler. It isn't as accurate, but it would help ease my mind. She found what we were pretty sure were three different heartbeats, and there was surely one right where the movement had stopped, in my upper left side.

The next morning I went to my appointment with only a little nagging worry. We went through the ultrasound and she scanned babies A and B as we chatted and asked questions, but by the time she had gotten to C, I had zoned out since I was so tired. Then she said she would be right back with the doctor. A minute later the doctor came and scanned in silence. I was afraid to ask questions for fear he would just say, "I'll get to that" or "I'm looking." So we had about 15 minutes where the doctor scanned the heartbeats, and no one said a word. It was torture. I knew there was something wrong, but I didn't know what it was and couldn't ask. Finally the doctor said, "Here's the thing…" He went on to explain that Baby A had way too much fluid, and Baby C had so little she was what they called "stuck on the top", above the other two babies. Additionally, she hadn't grown in the last 3 weeks. He showed me her heartbeat and although it didn't stop, it did something different. I was too out of it to know exactly what he was saying, though. He told me that he would call Seattle and set up an appointment for me, asking when I could get there. I looked at my mother in law, Nancy, who said, "Anytime. I know we are busy, but the babies are more important." I was honestly too out of it to think straight. Just then my husband called. I asked if there was any way he could call during the appointment because I didn't want to go without talking to him again, so I asked if I could leave for a second and stepped into the other room. At this point, what I had gathered about laser surgery was that I was risking all three of my babies to the point that I would most likely lose them. I asked Cody if there was any way he could be there during the surgery. He said he would check. Soon I was back in the doctor's room. He had already called the hospital in Seattle and left a message. He said they would call back and set up an appointment. It wasn't until the ultrasound tech said, "I think you're choosing to do the right thing," that I thought we had any other options; at this rate, the extra fluid was going to put me into labor soon.

By the end of the day, I knew I was going to Seattle - driving on Sunday, appointment on Monday, surgery on Tuesday, and going home on Wednesday. I got an email from the coordinator there with a full description of the procedure and all the risks etc. I forwarded it to my mom and sisters, then called my mom to talk about what it said. She was reading a lot of it aloud to everyone in the room, and when she got to the risks, I had to ask her to stop. I had already read them and I couldn't think about them again. It said the surgery was still considered a success even if I lost two of the babies, as long as I kept one. I found that even talking to family about the situation became hard. When Cody called me that night, it was so nice to talk to him, I realized, "OK, this isn't my problem; it is our problem."

For the next two days I was completely out of it. I had to reschedule a hair appointment, because I couldn't think enough to get someone to watch the kids and drive to it. Cody was always great when he called. I would be all worry, and he would say, "It's going to be ok." I always felt a little better after we talked. We decided that he wouldn't try and come home unless I went into labor or something, because he had stuff to get done so he could come home for good. Leaving before then meant having to start all over again. Plus, I wasn't sure if I could let him leave home again, knowing how miserable I was without him.

On Sunday, we drove to Seattle and on Monday went for the consultation. The ultrasound took 4 hours! We had originally decided to wait until Cody got back to find out the sexes together, but with everything I kept reading about people losing one or more of the babies, we decided to find out. I wanted my babies to have names if any of them didn't make it.

So we found out that our babies were girls. We tried to be light and get excited that I was going to have four girls under a year old. We discussed names and how life was going to be crazy, but the whole time I had that nagging fear that I may end up with just one. It was four days since my last ultrasound, and baby A was in heart failure. The doctor was more worried about baby A than C. She said I was in Stage 3.

Someone asked me, if it was necessary to kill one of the babies, would I? I just kept praying that God would save me from having to make that decision. In all the papers I had to sign, it never said the doctors could do whatever they thought best without my permission, but that was still something that I feared. I asked the doctor if she recommended termination of baby A, to save the others. She said no, that they would do whatever they could to save all of my babies, but that if, by chance, one of the babies didn't make it, by lasering shut the connections, the others wouldn't be affected. I was relieved, since it sounded like the doctor saw my babies' lives like I did: not something, but someone.

That night was so long. I texted Cody several times throughout the night to tell him I was scared. I knew I shouldn't, because it was so hard for him to be away from me, going insane from not knowing what was going to happen. Eliza was up all night, but that was fine since I couldn't sleep anyway. Plus, I was so thirsty and not allowed to drink; being pregnant with multiples and nursing, I got extremely thirsty.

The next morning I went for surgery. My blood pressure was high, but they said that was nor-

mal, everyone has high blood pressure before a surgery. I was coughing pretty badly so I asked if I could
get a nebulizer treatment first. I didn't want to cough
when the doctor was trying to laser something. My
sister, Maria, was there with me, along with Nancy,
who had been to every appointment. Maria is a
nurse, so it was very helpful to ask her "Is that normal?" about everything. She found it funny that I
was more worried about an IV and surgery than I was
about having five kids under 3. I had never had surgery, nor been in the hospital. I was scared of that
alone, the fear of losing my babies added on top.
Cody kept texting Maria and Nancy and it sounded
like he was panicking, too. It took them hours to prep
me and he was in Virginia, waiting, imagining the
worst. The surgery took about 50 minutes. They said
there were connections between all three babies. I got
to watch, and the doctor showed us baby B's face, her
hand, etc. It was really cool; she was only 18 weeks,
but looked fully developed since we could see little
fingernails and her tiny ear. She liked to move a lot
and it got frustrating for the doctors. They would be
ready to laser, when a foot would get right in the way.
When they finished lasering, they took 1.5 liters of
fluid from baby A's sac. I'm pretty sure I got smaller.
Afterwards, they kept me in the hospital overnight,
where they monitored for contractions and checked
my blood pressure.

My sister had Eliza with her, so I had my first
night without my baby. It really wasn't awful, but I
already felt so bad about leaving my son, Gareth. I
felt so guilty leaving my kids all the time, especially
with their dad already gone. Everyone said they
would be just fine, but I know it was hard on them.
Cody called Gareth, who just kept asking where his

mama and sister were. I had tried to tell him, but a 3 year old can only grasp so much.

I didn't have many contractions, and the next morning they did another ultrasound. The babies were looking a lot better, and baby A's heart was already healing. Babies A and B had more fluid, so the doctor was very happy and optimistic.

They sent me home with orders to see my doctor every week for four weeks. If something was going to go wrong, it would most likely happen within the first two weeks. The surgery didn't hurt much and I wasn't having contractions, but I was still sore for the eight hour drive home.

HOPE: Another ultrasound and the size difference was now 3 weeks 3 days. We no longer waited for the doctor to open the results; we opened them ourselves, and on this evening, rang Dr. C. at home to inform him the growth was falling further apart. He wanted us in his office at 10 the next morning to discuss our plan of attack. There, he announced we had an appointment with a top OB in Sydney (around a 6 hour drive) in two days' time. He believed what we were experiencing was consistent with a condition called Twin to Twin Transfusion Syndrome. This was something relatively unheard of in Australia, but the doctor in Sydney would talk to us more.

David went straight to work, jumping on the internet to research. Comparing the bits he found, what we had going on matched the symptoms of TTTS. He emailed a lady from one of the websites, asking for additional information.

In Sydney, we had another ultrasound, and it was at this time we learned that we were having girls; I was so excited about that. The growth difference was still showing at 3 weeks, 3 days. TTTS was discussed with us, but this particular doctor admitted he was not very well informed on this condition and that as far as he knew, there was really no one in Australia who had much knowledge of treatments for it. My fluid levels were just ok, so they decided to monitor me very closely and see what happened. We also had a consulted with a gene specialist, to put our minds slightly at ease regarding the suspected Downs Syndrome. She found that the chance of one of the babies carrying such a disorder was 1 in 988,000. We were offered an amnio, but I decided the risk of miscarriage was too high for me, so I refused.

Upon arriving home that night, I found a Fed Ex package at our front door. Weird - I wasn't expecting anything. I opened it up to find a binder full of info and stories on TTTS; the kind lady (I sadly admit, I cannot remember her name) had posted this parcel from America for us to read. It contained the story of how she lost her babies, plus info on treatment-- everything we could possibly want. After reading it, I was convinced that this was what was going on. I had the symptoms, but now I also had some knowledge of what might or might not happen.

WRIGHT: Another week where everything stayed stable! The doctors were starting to talk about when I reached 24 weeks; they could take my babies and try to save both of them in the NICU. They told me that if I made it, we would schedule the C-section, and I would quite possibly go home with both of my girls.

BRAY: By week 18, I started to feel very uncomfortable. My stomach was very big. I had very bad back pain and felt a lot of pressure down below. I thought to myself, "How the hell am I meant to carry on working for another 15 weeks?" I wasn't even halfway through my pregnancy, but felt as though I could give birth at any second. I knew something wasn't right. I was also concerned that I had not yet felt the babies kick. I had an appointment for a scan in two weeks, but decided to ring the antenatal clinic and ask their advice. I spoke to a midwife, who explained that I would need to go through the ante natal inpatient ward. I was put through to the ward. I explained that I was at 18 weeks gestation, and carrying twins. She asked what the problem was, so I explained all the symptoms I was having. She told me that because I was only at 18 weeks, they wouldn't "deal" with me on the ward, and that I had to ring my local doctor. By this time, it was late evening and my local office was closed, so I rang the out of hours service. I was seen that evening by my general practitioner, who told me he thought I had a water infection, and that I should take some antibiotics and wait for my 20 week scan. I went home knowing full well I didn't have a water infection, so I signed off work on the sick and waited for my scan appointment.

FLETCHER: I made an appointment to see Dr. B., as I had had another ultrasound and lost a lot of fluid during that time period. When Pam did the ultrasound, I remember looking in horror; there was hardly any fluid. Abby was lying on top of Ally. Again I thought, this is it, my babies are gone. But God had other things in store for us. He had far bigger plans than we could ever have IMAGINED. I remember Pam crying, and having to see Dr. A. that day. After talking with her, I felt I had taken all I could, emotionally. As we were leaving, he wrote the word "abortion" on my file. It was a "natural abortion", as she called it. That word would stick in my head forever! I thought, "I am not aborting this pregnancy." So why did she write that word on my file? Then I realized what she meant. We would just keep a closer eye on Ally and Abby from there on out.

DOBBS: On August 25, 2005, we found out that we would be having girls, and that one of them was 10 oz. and the other one was 7.9 oz. The doctor said my due date was around January 24, 2006. It still had not yet sunk in that we were having twins.

13
Week 19

BRUCH: Within seven days of diagnosis, we found ourselves at the Children's Hospital of Philadelphia (CHOP). After a long day of tests, ultrasounds, and doctors poking and prodding, we received terrible news. The boys had a 30% size difference between them. On the TTTS scale our boys were a two. We were given five options. One was to terminate, killing both. The second was to sacrifice one in hope the other would survive. Third, try laser surgery. Fourth, try amnio reductions. Fifth, do nothing and lose both in a matter of weeks. We wanted them ; we were there for two babies. We could barely wrap our heads around these choices, but we had to decide. If we did nothing, we would lose both in a matter of weeks. We were just crushed. I will never forget that conversation.

HADDIGAN: Our surgery went well, and we were able to see our recipient onscreen during the procedure. They removed three liters of fluid. Both twins were doing well immediately following the surgery, but that night seemed like forever. The next day, after another ultrasound, our recipient's bladder was seen - finally! Their fluid levels were close to even, and things were finally looking good. We stayed another night, and the following day the ultrasound was great! Both boys looked wonderful and we were sent home.

SLICHTER: During my 19th week of pregnancy, our world came crashing down. Since Jack had such a slim chance of survival, we made the extremely hard decision to terminate him to save Jake. The specialist assured us that at least we would have one healthy baby. So one week before my 20th birthday, we decided to have the selective reduction laser surgery. The procedure was scheduled for a Wednesday. On Tuesday, I received a call from the hospital, telling me that my insurance would not cover it. It was quite an expensive surgery that my husband and I would not be able to afford without insurance. According to Tricare, they could not approve the $13,000 procedure, because it was technically an abortion. I was overly stressed by the insurance company that week, but finally, on Thursday, I got the call from the hospital that the doctors had proved it medically necessary and insurance had approved it - two days after my scheduled appointment!

I went in on Friday for the procedure. Before I could be wheeled into surgery, they had to do another ultrasound, to figure out where to go in. Unfortunately, Jack had already passed. I burst into tears, and even the nurses with me were crying. It was a very sad day.

Now, the focus was on Jake. I went for another ultrasound later, and the specialist said that Jake already showed signs of brain failure. We went home; it was a long, quiet drive. We were both upset and confused. We didn't know what to do.

CADLE: During week 19, I called my doctor and told them what the specialist had said. He finally agreed to see me. That was when my life changed forever. I went by myself, since Ronnie worked an hour away. I just thought the doctor was just going to tell me something simple, that everything would be okay, but

that's not how it turned out. When I got there, my
B.P. was 142/72, and I had lost 4 pounds. I knew then
that something was not right and I was freaking out!
The doctor examined me and said that my cervix was
closed and that everything seemed fine. He then tried
to hear their heartbeats, but there were none. He
called the office where I had had my first and only
sonogram, and got me an appointment for right then.
I had the same tech, and she started scanning. It
showed my babies just lying there, no movement, no
heartbeats, nothing. They were gone, all three of
them.

This is what the report said:

"Triplet gestation with no fetal heart tones.
Previously reported fetus, which appeared to be deformed with no heart activity, labeled Fetus C, was
not seen on this examination. Fetuses A and B were
seen; there appeared to be deformity of the bones of
the cranium, therefore no weight or measurements
could be obtained. There was no fetal heart activity
for fetus A or B."

The tech asked if I was alone. I said yes, so she
asked, "Can I call someone for you?" I gave her my
phone and had her call Ronnie. I drove home and
waited for Ronnie to arrive. I was in shock and could
not believe they were gone. I called my mom and dad
,and waited to hear from my doctor. He got me an
appointment with a specialist. There, they told me
that my boys were dead, and that it appeared to be
TTTS. This is the one and only time we were told
anything like TTTS had been wrong. We were left
hanging for weeks, waiting and wanting to know
why our babies had died. They kept saying that

Drake, baby C, had died from something else and kind of made it out that he had never really existed at all.

Here is what the specialists found:

- Triplet gestation with no fetal heart tones

- Fetal hydrops is present

- Placenta location-posterior/left lateral

- Amniotic fluid volume is consistent with oligohydraminos in Sac C

- Triplet A is 15 6/7 weeks gest. Age

- Triplet B is 14 5/7 weeks gest. age

- Triplet C is 10 1/7 weeks gest. age

- Placenta x2 appear to be fused

- Triamniotic /Dichorionic triplet gest.

- Triplet A and B appear to have been Diamniotic-Monochorionic twins with TTTS

- Amniotic fluid volume for triplet A is consistent with polyhydraminos in Sac A

- Amniotic fluid volume for triplet B is consistent with oligohydraminos in Sac B

- Amniotic fluid volume for triplet C is consistent with oligohydraminos in Sac C

- No FHT's were found, consistent with intrauterine fetal demise in triplet C

- Triplet C appears to have been possible anencephalic with scoliosis or possible rachischisis.

This was mortifying. How could any mother

read this and figure out what had happened? How could these terms help a mother understand this disease?

<u>MARTIN:</u> The OB said I had to get detailed ultrasounds by the hospital every appointment. During a few previous ultrasounds, the doctor had told us that one twin was measuring a few weeks ahead of the other. We had no idea that anything could be wrong. We thought this was normal, no cause for alarm, or at least that's the way we took it from our doctor. After a new ultrasound at the hospital, we were told that one twin was a boy, so we assumed the other was also. At that time we were told that they were in the same corion, but in different sacs and sharing one placenta. The doctor told me that I needed an appointment in Galveston, for a high resolution ultrasound. We headed out a few days later, thinking that we'd make a day of it. I love Galveston; it was my getaway when I was in high school, and we go sometimes just to breathe. We left my daughter with my mom, which turned out to be a good thing.

After our ultrasound, the waiting lasted forever. The doctor finally came in and gave us three choices. 1 - several amniocenteses, 2 - laser surgery a.k.a. placental ablation, 3 - tie off one to save the other. Then he told me why - TTTS STAGE 4! Out of 5 stages, we were in LATE stage 4. How could we miss this? How could this happen? Did we do anything wrong? All these questions popped into our heads. Our lives were over.

The doctor was surprised the babies were still alive. Evan, we later named him, had all the fluid, around his belly, head, and heart. Ethan had none.

Our poor baby looked dried up. Ethan was so little compared to Evan. Ethan was called the Donor twin, while Evan was the Recipient. Ethan's sac was barely there, no bladder was visible, and it was a horrible sight. We measured our odds, after we broke down. We only had seconds to decide the fate of our children, not knowing if one option was better than the other, having NEVER been educated on such a disease. We didn't know WHAT to do. After talking with the doctor, option 3 was not for us. Saving one or the other was GOD'S choice; we didn't feel right trying to "play God" so to speak. We decided on option 2, the surgery, after we were told that amniotic reductions might not be successful, but would be painful. The chances with the laser were somewhat better, and we hoped that we could at least give our boys a little bit of a fighting chance.

We needed to act fast, so they set us up in Houston for the next morning. My mother-in-law insisted we stay in a Houston hotel. We took the long and emotionally painful drive back to Vidor to see my daughter before we left, not knowing what was going to happen to me or the babies. After a quick "I love you", we packed our bags and headed to Houston, only to find that my mother-in-law's "awesome" plans had fallen through.

We had no choice but to stay at her house in Pearland. My husband and I just wanted time alone, and we were not able to have that. We were both scared, not knowing if the babies and I would be okay. But we couldn't even sleep in the same bed, since she didn't have one big enough for us. That was the worst night. I needed my husband by my side, not having to entertain others, at this point in my life.

TUMMERS: My appointment this week was with someone different, due to scheduling issues. The doctor I saw was female, and great. She did a thorough scan and said all looked well. I had gained the most weight I'd yet gained…a whopping five pounds in two weeks! I asked about this, but she said it wasn't a concern. I also asked her about my babies being more than a week apart in growth, but she told me it is only of concern if there is more than a 25% difference. She looked briefly at the results of my scan from the week before, and reported that everything looked fine.

LIGHT: I was gaining weight fast, and started wondering if something was wrong when, in one week, I gained over 8lbs!

On February 22nd (at 26 weeks gestation), after the ultrasound that revealed we were having identical boys, I received instructions from the radiologist to call Triage at Grand River Hospital because there was a problem with the scan. Without really thinking, we rushed out the door to the hospital. There, we were told that there was a possibility we had Twin-To-Twin Transfusion Syndrome.

We were referred to Dr. Gregory Ryan; The Director of Fetal Medicine at Mount Sinai Hospital, in Toronto Ontario. After a quick assessment, he sat us down and told us the boys were definitely suffering from TTTS, as well as from a rare condition called Growth Discordance. We were between stages 2 and 3, and treatment was necessary for their survival. We were given a few options:
A) Endoscopic Laser surgery with amnioreduction
B) Amnioreduction

C) Elective Termination of the Donor
D) Do nothing

We chose a treatment based on statistics, which treatment's outcome was the most optimistic, as well as what the Doctor suggested. My husband was the one who asked all the appropriate questions, especially the ones that I was most afraid of.

CHRISTMAN-SCHARER: I had my next appointment with the perinatologists a few days later. Dr. F. did a Level II ultrasound that took two hours. It still showed the very early stages of TTTS. They wanted me to go to CHOP by the end of the week, to see a specialist. The babies were growing well and they looked good. Twin A had less fluid, but her bladder was showing. Twin B had a lot of fluid. The babies weighed 11 oz. and 13 oz. I was having a hard time sleeping or getting comfortable now. My feet hurt a lot as well.

MORGAN: This was the second scariest appointment we experienced. The fluid levels had changed for the worse. We were instructed to wait while the doctor called a laser surgery specialist in Bellevue, WA. We had two days to fly up there and have the surgery, or we would lose both of our babies. In Bellevue, the babies were examined by ultrasound. They were at Stage IV. My back throbbed and I was very bloated.

We had the procedure done on a Friday afternoon. On Saturday, they wheeled me down to check on the babies, and see how they had responded to the surgery. During the ultrasound, the doctor turned to me and said, "I'm sorry…there is no heartbeat in baby B. I am sorry."

My husband and I were silent... we were stiff as boards. We had not been expecting it to turn out this way. As I was wheeled back up to my hospital room, I lost it. I tried to be strong and hold back my tears, but I couldn't. I could not believe this was happening.

JELLEY: The day after coming home, I got really worried. I didn't feel any movement and I became paranoid. I called my mom, who called my OB, to see if she could get me a quick ultrasound. It turned out that she wasn't doing office visits that day, just meetings, but she said she could do a quick one on her lunch break. Right away, I could see movement on the scan. Although it was a little sad that I couldn't feel the movement, it really set my mind at ease that they were moving. There were still three heartbeats, and although it was a really quick look, it was obvious that baby C had fluid.

WRIGHT: It really seemed as though the bed rest and protein shakes were working! My girls were moving all the time. I began to feel a little more relaxed about going to my appointments. There was still about a 20% disparity between my girls, but they were both growing and the fluid levels staying about the same.

DILLE: We had a regular check up on the morning of November 7th, 2008. I had some concerns about weight, gaining over 10 pounds during the previous week or so. I thought it might be just the twin pregnancy, or maybe that I was developing gestational diabetes. My doctor checked me over and did a quick ultrasound. She said the babies looked okay, but that I did have quite a bit of fluid. She seemed unconcerned about that, since I was pregnant with twins.

My regular ultrasound was scheduled for later that afternoon. I came back with my husband and my mom. We were all so excited to check on the babies, and to find out if we were having two boys, two girls, or one of each. The ultrasound tech started scanning and we could tell fairly early on that something wasn't quite right. Baby A was swimming all over the place while Baby B was barely able to move at all. The tech looked for the dividing membrane, but it was so thin that it took close to 20 minutes to find. Then, my husband started asking questions about why Baby B wasn't moving. The tech wouldn't really answer him, though. She scanned what she could and got what measurements she could. She was able to determine the sex of the babies. We were having girls! I was so excited; I was going to get the twin baby girls I had always wanted.

My excitement was soon shattered when the tech went to get a doctor to speak with us. He was not my regular doctor, but the only doctor there that late Friday afternoon. He told us that our girls had something called TTTS. I had read about this condition briefly in my pregnancy book, but didn't know too many details about it. The doctor explained to us what TTTS was - that the babies did not have an equal share of the placenta. He said that Baby B was basically shrink-wrapped, and that Baby A had all of the fluid in her sac. We did have some options available to us, including laser ablation surgery, which was done in only a handful of hospitals across the United States. We were informed that if we did nothing to treat this condition, the chance we would lose both baby girls was greater than a 90%. We needed an appointment with a specialist right away.

We left the office very emotional, not knowing what our future held. When we got home, we did as much online research about TTTS as we could. We also started choosing names. I wanted my baby girls to have their own names, right away, in case something was to happen to them. The names we chose were Cara Grace and Tessa Anne.

My husband and I went to see the specialist that Monday, and they confirmed the diagnosis of TTTS. I believe we were at stage 2 at that point. Cara, the donor twin, had a barely visible bladder. There wasn't a huge size difference, but it was enough to be an issue. We were advised to make the appointment for a surgical consultation for later that week. We drove three hours to Seattle, Washington, to meet with the doctors there. My husband had to stay home with a very sick toddler, so my dad drove. The diagnosis was confirmed again, and our stage had not changed. I had a ton of extra fluid; though I don't remember the fluid pocket levels, I think they were around 15 centimeters. Cara had less than 1. The girls appeared to be fairly healthy despite the diagnosis, so we weren't yet candidates for the surgery. I was sent home on modified bed rest.

FLETCHER: I had to see Dr. B. every two weeks, and Dr. L. every week, until the day I would deliver. I remember going that next week, thinking, "They are going to tell me both girls are gone." Erin started the ultrasound and did all of her things before the doctor came in. I told him everything that Dr. Q. had told us. I didn't want to look at the screen, but when I did, they had fluid again! God had answered a prayer. Ally's head would be stuck in the birth canal until I delivered, which is how they kept their fluid. I would sit out on our deck and see these two birds, always flying together. They never left each other's side. I thought this was a sign from God. Our girls were going to be ok.

DOBBS: August 31, 2005, my thyroid was in normal range and I would not need to go back to Dr. F.

BRUCE: On July 6, 2007, at 19 weeks 5 days gestation, we went for an ultrasound with the Maternal Fetal Medicine doctor. The ultrasound tech and doctor said very little to us about the status of our girls. We still knew little about TTTS or even what questions to ask.

14
Week 20

BRUCH: We chose laser surgery. We were told that they might not be able to do anything; the placenta being located on my belly made it very difficult to even get the scope in. If they could, would they see what they needed to save my sons? We were helpless, but figured we had to act in some way.

HADDIGAN: After bed rest, I was given the ok to return to work. Our OB referred us to the specialist due to our high-risk pregnancy. I didn't want to meet all new doctors; I liked the doctor I had. Things were looking good on ultrasound. We picked out our names: Riley William and Logan Edward. Finally, it looked like our boys were going to beat the odds.

SLICHTER: In my 20th week, we went back to the local high-risk specialist. The doctor conducted an ultrasound and said that he did not see anything at all wrong with Jake's brain. We were very confused, but hopeful that our son would be ok. I felt that we needed other opinions, so I made an appointment with another doctor for the following week

MARTIN: It was not definite that we would have surgery, so we had no idea what was in store for us. After ANOTHER LONG ultrasound, they decided that we needed to have the surgery after all, and sent us to prep. Ours was the worst stage 4 they had ever seen. To the medical team, we were the "new experiment". They were truly nice and caring, though. They held our hand the whole time and truly made us feel at home. These people had practiced this surgery around the world. They were the best.

We were advised that both babies could die by simply entering the uterus, which was made to hold and not to be punctured, even with the rice grain size needle that would be inserted. But they didn't. The amniotic fluid was nasty due to the previous clot, which was nowhere to be found, so they removed it. That should have put them into shock, but our boys were troopers! I lost 10 pounds of fluid alone. After the procedure was done, there were still two heart-beats. I was snoring so loudly that the doctors had a hard time concentrating, and had to wake me up a bit. I hadn't been getting any sleep and I felt so relaxed, for the first time in a long time.

The first 24 hours would tell. There were two heart beats. Same at 48 hours. We were so excited that everything was PERFECT. Strict bed rest was ordered. Our hopes were so high. We still had some time to wait and see if everything was going to be okay, and I would have to make it to Houston once a week until the twins delivered. My husband stocked the fridge so my daughter could help herself; that way I could stay on the couch. My family shopped for groceries for me and brought me things to help me stay sane, while my husband returned to work. Through all of our problems, they continued to pay him for 40 hours, even if he wasn't at work.

After some time, I start leaking some type of fluid. In a panic, I called, scared to have to go BACK to Houston. I was told to see my local OB for an ultrasound, to check the fluids. At that ultrasound, they told me I had nothing to worry about, that the fluid was good and the small baby was doing very well. I was just urinating on myself due to the pressure from the babies.

TUMMERS: My anatomy scan took FOREVER! I was so uncomfortable through the whole 2 hour procedure. The tech asked me about how old my other boys were, so I assumed I was having boys. She told me that would be in the report to my doctor. I got great a picture of the babies… Baby B was sucking its thumb.

I felt crummy the rest of the week, and noticed that I just couldn't do things like climb stairs, etc. It was just too exhausting!

CHRISTMAN-SCHARER: When I was 20 weeks, I had my first appointment at CHOP. I had a level II ultrasound and a fetal echocardiogram. They assessed it as more of a placental deficiency than TTTS, but if it was TTTS, then it was very early stage. My placenta was not very good on Baby A's side. They were not sure why I had a placental deficiency. Twin A was stuck, with a small bladder and very little room, since she was the donor baby. Twin B, the recipient, had a large amount of fluid and a lot of room to move. Their sizes were good, but I had to go back in a week. They were trying to hold off ordering bed rest until I was about 24 weeks, because of my other children. I continued to work through the majority of this. I must have been insane. After I was told that I might need bed rest, we tried to find me some help around the house.

MORGAN: Back at Phoenix Perinatal, the doctor and nurses were so supportive. We were instructed to go twice a week for ultrasounds, to see the progress in the donor baby, Jadon. Though he had originally had no fluid around him and no bladder was visible, he beat the odds and began to thrive.

JELLEY: At 20 weeks, we went to see the doctor again. I was pretty worried; I kept saying I wished I could have an ultrasound every day. When we got there, I told the ultrasound tech, "I just want to see three heartbeats," and sure enough, there were still three heartbeats! The babies all looked great. Baby A's heart was still showing side effects from over-work, but it looked better. Baby C had fluid and was still growing. They said she would probably be be-hind in size until birth, but that as long as she kept growing, we didn't have to worry; she would catch up after she was born. Although she had fluid, her bladder still wasn't visible. No one seemed worried, though. It was a good, optimistic appointment.

BENNER: By 20 weeks, I was at stage 3. Mason's heart was beating faster, because of all the fluid he had to pump. Isiah's heart wasn't pumping blood like it should. Both had urine in their bladders.

HOPE: I have to admit, for the next eight weeks or so, things became a bit of a blur. We had countless ultrasounds, measuring growth and fluid. I was ad-mitted to the hospital several times, as I had devel-oped postural drop syndrome. (At any time, I could faint and fall flat on my stomach, which always led to a visit to the hospital for monitoring of heartbeats.) I never relaxed for one moment in these weeks. I still didn't enjoy being pregnant, didn't want to talk about it, and didn't want to see anyone. My life consisted of bed rest and trying to keep brave for myself, David, and my little girls. By this time, we had named both girls, so Twin A became Chloe, and Twin B became Jorja. I was such a regular at the hospital, and with my OB, that they all referred to my girls by their names, and no longer as A and B. I found this comforting. To me, it showed that these people cared and wanted to see my two little girls survive.

WRIGHT: At that week's ultrasound, I found out that my little Sarah had passed. After so many ultrasounds, I had gotten pretty good at understanding what I was looking at on the monitor. As soon as the technician scanned over her, I knew something was wrong. The tech hurriedly scanned Julie Anne, gave me a hug, and left the room. I called my husband overseas as I sat in the ultrasound room, but I could barely talk. All I could do was cry. He knew immediately what had happened. I was taken into another room, where the doctor came in to talk to me. He said that on the ultrasound, it looked like Sarah had just died, and that it appeared Julie Anne was in distress. Her heart rate was down, and her fluid level had dropped from 6.5dvp to 1.7dvp. He was almost certain that Julie Anne would die within the next 24 hours. He said to come back the next week, but I told him I'd be back in 25 hours for a re-scan. He agreed, and amazingly, she was still alive!

DILLE: Two days after my appointment in Seattle, I felt as though things were getting worse. I was in so much pain that I could barely move. My ribs were being spread apart by the increasing levels of fluid. I called Dr. W. in Seattle, who told me to come in the next morning, a Sunday. An ultrasound showed the girls' condition had become a little worse (I believe we were at a stage 3), which made us eligible for the surgery. The OR wasn't available Monday, so my surgery was scheduled for Tuesday morning. I felt such relief; I was going to be able to save my babies!

I don't remember much from the surgery, except that I felt like I couldn't breathe. I think I slept through most of it. After it was over, the surgeons reported finding and treating about 15 shared blood vessels, and that the girls had about a 60 / 40 split of the placenta. They had drained a little over three liters of fluid from Tessa. The surgery was considered a success and they were very optimistic about the survival of both girls. The next 18 hours were spent in bed, on terbutiline to control the contractions caused by the surgery. I felt tons of baby movement all through the night, which I thought was a positive sign, but I was having terrible pain in my legs from the anesthetic, and I was nervous that I might go into pre-term labor.

I was taken for an ultrasound early the next morning. I was still nervous, but truly felt like I had saved my babies and everything was going to be fine. However, when the nurse started the scan and then called for the doctor right away, my husband and I knew immediately that something was wrong. The doctor scanned me for a second, and then told us that he was sorry, but Tessa had not made it through the night. I was in complete shock, just disbelief. I didn't even cry. When I left to go to the bathroom before continuing the exam, the doctor asked my husband if I was okay. My husband told him that I would probably break down and cry when we got back to our room, away from other people. And that is exactly what I did. My parents were at the hospital watching my two older children. When they called to ask how things were going, we had to tell them one of their granddaughters had died. They told my son, Tyler (6), that one of his baby sisters had died. My youngest, Caylee, was too young to understand. The only thing she knew was that Mommy had babies in her belly, because she would point to my belly and say, "Babies!"

We had another ultrasound later that afternoon, to check on Cara. I was petrified to be wheeled into the exam room, but was soon relieved to hear that Cara was doing well. She had a strong heartbeat and was already gaining fluid. We stayed in the hospital another night, and had one more ultrasound the next morning. Cara was alive, and her condition had improved some more, so we were discharged from the hospital. We were told to follow up with our high-risk pregnancy clinic at home once a week, for detailed ultrasounds to monitor Cara. And so we went home, confused and sad.

BRAY: I was 20 weeks and 4 days gestation on March 17. I lay on the bed as the nurse began the scan. I could see the concern in her eyes. "Are there two heartbeats?" I asked. "Are my babies ok?" She made no eye contact with me, but said, "Yes, there are two heartbeats". "Are they ok?" I repeated. She looked at me, and asked if I had been told whether or not the babies were in individual sacs. "Yes," I answered, "They had to do an internal to double check." But she defiantly told me the babies didn't have their own sacs. Then she explained that she could not see the membrane. She also informed us that she was finding it very difficult to perform the scan, as I was carrying very large amounts of amniotic fluid. She contacted a consultant radiologist, saying, "He will be able to see what is going on with your twins." So I was taken to the radiology department, where I saw Dr. D., who confirmed that we had TTTS. We had, as he put it, "stuck twin syndrome." The scan had shown that our donor twin had little or no amniotic fluid, was shrink-wrapped in his amniotic sac, and had no visible bladder. He was very sick. Dr. D. went on to tell us that our recipient twin was in massive amounts of amniotic fluid. He told us that he was no expert in this condition, and would refer us to a more appropriate doctor. But our local hospital had very little knowledge about TTTS, so we were referred to a doctor at St. Michael's Hospital, in Bristol, England.

OROSZ: I had gotten regular scans until week 20, when I cancelled my ultrasound appointment due to weather.

BRUCE: Since my doctors, tight-lipped during appointments, were doing very little to help us, I took it upon myself to research TTTS on the internet. On July 9, 2007, at 20 weeks gestation, I contacted a TTTS specialist referenced in many online articles. I told the specialist everything my Maternal Fetal Medicine doctor had explained to us about the condition of our twins. The specialist stated that, based on what I had told him, the twins seemed to be doing okay, but that I should start asking during each ultrasound: how much fluid was in each twins' sac? How much did each twin weigh? What did my cervix measure? And lastly, what was the percentage of discord between the twins? He also suggested that I drink Ensure or Boost protein shakes, to put weight on the twins in case early delivery was necessary.

15
Week 21

<u>BRUCH:</u> They ultimately couldn't complete the laser surgery due to the anterior placenta. They removed 3.66 liters of fluid from the recipient's amniotic sac, but were only able to see the recipient's cord. They could not even see where the placenta started on the donor baby, much less his cord insertion. All we could try was amnio reductions, or selecting the recipient baby be killed, in hope that the donor would survive. The doctors gave us time to make the decision. Four days after the surgery, at our final visit to CHOP, our donor baby was 40% smaller than the recipient baby. We were still a 2 on the Quintero stage. We just couldn't choose to kill the "sicker" baby. He was our son, and we believed, as parents, that we needed to protect our child no matter what. Even if we did terminate him, the other could die anyway. Could we live with ourselves, knowing they might both have made had we had just let them be?

<u>HADDIGAN:</u> Week 21 I had some leaking. The OB checked things out and said that everything looked ok, but to rest in bed over the weekend.

<u>SLICHTER:</u> The following week, we met with another good doctor to get her opinion about my pregnancy. She said that everything looked good. She, too, did not see anything wrong with Jake's brain. I wanted yet another opinion, so she referred me to another doctor. Two days later, I was in his office getting an ultrasound, and he saw nothing wrong, either. We were so confused - why were the doctors saying different things? We were lost, and there wasn't much

we felt we could do. I kept my appointment with the high-risk doctor for the following week.

TUMMERS: My regular OB saw me that week and reported that everything looked great on the ultrasound… no concerns at all. The tech had NOT put the sex in the report, and our doctor said it was important for him to know this, to confirm that all was as he thought. To this day, I am not sure what that meant. It was obvious that I was carrying monochorionic twins, given their concern about the dividing membrane, but each ultrasound, either questioned or reconfirmed this. One tech would see the membrane and the next wouldn't. The doctor scanned me again, and my babies were super active, especially baby A -- kicking baby B in the head! All looked great, according to my doctor. He couldn't determine the sex after all, but said he'd guess girls.

We spoke about my weight, as I'd gained none in the last two weeks. He wasn't concerned about that, as long as I was eating well. I was still seeing the dietician that had helped me lose weight, and she was keeping me focused on healthy eating.

LIGHT: We chose endoscopic laser surgery, and amnioreductions, knowing that was the option with the most optimistic results, though even after the surgery, the Recipient (Sebastian) had a 54% chance of survival, and the Donor (Oliver) had a 26% chance, with a 36% chance both would survive. We agreed to the surgery without hesitation.

On February 26th, I was under the OR lights at Mt. Sinai, the lives of our babies in the careful hands of Doctor R. Rob sat right next to me the whole time, and was able to see the babies: "Little Oli, all wrapped up in the separating membrane, like a kid behind a shower curtain trying to look through. His big brother Seb, just free floating away, kicking and hitting the probe as it moves around him."

A few days after the surgery, Dr. R. gave us the OK to go home, but made sure we were aware that we weren't out of the woods yet. Oliver was still very little (not even big enough to be on the size charts), but he did have a much better chance now. Once at home, we went for weekly ultrasounds, with every other week done by Dr. R. at Mount Sinai. Both babies were growing, but especially Sebastian! Oliver was slowly but surely increasing in size, but he was still dangerously small. Still, we kept our hopes up for him, silently aware of the possibility of only having Sebastian.

CHRISTMAN-SCHARER: We went back to CHOP, at 21 weeks. They still thought it was more of a placental deficiency than TTTS. I had to go back in 2 weeks. The doctor said the girls looked good, and I felt them moving a lot. My side and belly hurt by the end of the day. I was having trouble sleeping, and became out of breath easily, so I went to the local doctor for a scan. He said the babies were doing well, but Twin A was stuck and I definitely had a placental issue and TTTS. Then I went to my regular ob-gyn to do a 24-hour urine test for preeclampsia, because my blood pressure was up.

REBILAS: I was finally diagnosed with TTTS. The Donor was 10oz and Recipient was 16oz. I was put on bed rest immediately. This didn't work out too well, as we had just bought a new home! I contacted the TTTS Foundation and they overnighted me a packet, which included their binder full of knowledge! I was overwhelmed but felt a little more prepared. I contacted Dr. D. of Wisconsin, who called me personally the next day. He told me that I could "help" myself by drinking Ensure and adhering to strict bed rest. It didn't seem like much, but I was willing to do what I had to do. The hardest part was that I had a 2 year old running around the house. My mother in law would come over to help with our son by making him lunch. He would bring me books and we would sit and read. There was a lot of cuddling time. I tried to stay off of the computer, because of the sad stories I read. I wanted to stay positive!

JELLEY: That week went very well. Baby C had a visible bladder now, all three babies were growing at the same pace, and had the same amount of fluid.

BENNER: We went back to stage 2! YEAH!

OROSZ: I rescheduled my ultrasound for 21 weeks. Baby B (donor) was showing signs of TTTS, with low amniotic fluid compared to baby A (recipient). The doctor told me to drink Boost or Ensure three times a day, and to come back in a week to scan for improvement. I got in touch with the TTTS Foundation.

I had feared TTTS in my pregnancy, even before the new doctor told me about it. I had bought books on twins and looked up identical twins on the net. Getting TTTS was my worst fear, because I had read all the risks, and stories of loss. I was so afraid of that happening to me; when we were told we had TTTS, it was surreal. I wanted it to be a dream so badly, but instead it was my worst nightmare come true. I had never imagined getting pregnant with identical twins, let alone ending up in the 15% of identical twins with the disease! I could barely move. My stomach hurt so badly, it felt like I was stretched to the max.

DOBBS: September 14, 2005, I started spotting and called the doctor. He said bed rest the rest of the day and he'd see me first thing in the morning. September 15, I had lots of cramping. I was due to go to the doctor for my spotting, but he advised me to stay on bed rest for the rest of the week, with my feet up. He said I was over doing it.

DILLE: My husband and I went to the high-risk clinic for our first appointment after losing Tessa. I was so nervous that something was going to happen to Cara. The tech knew about our loss, so I specifically asked her not to scan Tessa, because it was too upsetting. I regret that some now. I wish I'd had more chances to look at her. I wish I had sought a 3D scan immediately after we lost her, so I would have that picture.

The ultrasound tech and the doctor were very concerned about me. I wasn't showing much emotion, but was very obviously depressed. It angered me when the nurse spoke to the doctor about my demeanor. I thought to myself, "Why shouldn't I be depressed? I just lost my baby girl." (I know now that their concern was genuine, for me, and for the loss that I had suffered.) The doctor gave us the results. He said that Cara did have some edema, a little water on her heart and in her body, but that this was normal given what she had been through. They would continue to monitor her the following week. Her Dopplers were all normal, and she had no signs of hydrops. We left, still concerned for our survivor.

16
Week 22

BRUCH: We had a conscious amnio reduction. They took two liters this time. On the Quintero stage, we were still a 2. The amnio reductions were so painful; as they drained the fluid, they began to move and kick. So as my uterus was contracting, they were trying to take up more room. It felt as if I was in labor, and I thought to myself, "Could I be losing both now?" I was put in a room to track my contractions, where I stayed until they stopped. Thank God, my sons were still ALIVE!

HADDIGAN: Week 22, bleeding! No contractions, but the OB told us to go to the hospital and get checked. Everything seemed fine and we were sent home for more bed rest.

SLICHTER: During this appointment with my high-risk doctor, he noticed that something was wrong. He said Jake had developed hydrops around his brain, heart, and organs. He said that even if Jake made it to birth, he would most likely have to be on a feeding tube. He wouldn't be able to walk or talk, and there was a good chance he wouldn't make it to his first birthday. We were given the option to continue the pregnancy, or to terminate. Although some may not agree, we felt that this type of life was not what we wanted for our child, that it wasn't much of a life at all. So, together we made the decision to terminate Jake. In our hearts, we felt it was the best option, and in his best interest. We would meet with another doctor at UNC the following week.

MARTIN: The next Wednesday (and every Wednes-day), I was supposed to go to Houston. The babies were not expected to make it that long. We were told, and saw for ourselves, that the membranes had sepa-rated. They maintained that I was urinating on my-self.

The Friday after that appointment, I was in the bathtub, against my husband's will. It had been a stressful few weeks, and I JUST wanted to relax in the tub. I even made sure the water wasn't hot, even though I love the hot water. At first, I thought the ba-bies didn't like the way I was sitting in the tub, which I barely fit into. I hadn't gone into labor with Emilee, so I didn't know what it felt like. There was none of the back pain I was forewarned about. The pains started off at 8pm, every 2 minutes, and only got worse. By 1:30am, my complaining woke my hus-band. I was up and down off the bed, looking into my pregnancy books and hoping they could tell me what was going on. I tried to get into the fetal posi-tion, on my knees, to TRY to sleep. I was so tired. My husband told me that I never complain about any-thing, and he was worried.

We headed to the hospital around 3am, after we dropped my daughter off at my grandmothers. My husband was literally going 100mph, hoping that a cop would pull us over and escort us to the hospital. No such luck. When we got there, I was fully dilated. They had already put the monitors on me when they realized this. The staff there was so nice and under-standing. They brought me to labor and delivery, and no more than five minutes later (while they were still getting ready), for some reason I pushed, and felt something come out. I told the nurse, but she said it was nothing. I pushed again, and as my husband turned to look at me, he saw a baby come out, then another on the next push. He was crying hysterically. It was his birthday and he saw EVERYTHING.

I have a heart condition, WPW (wolfe parkinson white). My heart has an extra pathway, and beats irregularly sometimes. Well, after I delivered the placenta, my pulse went up to nearly 190. My body started shaking and my bones wouldn't stop; I guess I was going in shock. I couldn't catch my breath, and since I'm kind of claustrophobic, the oxygen mask wasn't helping. I couldn't even think about the babies. I feel so guilty, even today, that I didn't think about them after they were born. I heard no cries, nothing. I don't even recall the group of people there to help our boys. The doctor had given me valium; I don't remember anything after that. My husband tells me that I was awake, or that at least my eyes were open, and that at that time, he was more worried about me. He thought he was going to lose me, too. Ethan died 30 minutes before I came to, and Evan was stillborn, though to this day, I don't believe it. I wish I could have seen them trying to save them, if they did so.

A really nice lady from NICU came in and asked me if I wanted pictures of the babies. This was all new to me, so I didn't know how to react. She told me that other women did it, since it would be all they had of their babies. So I agreed. I even took some pictures with them. I didn't know what kind of face to make for the pictures, so I just bit my bottom lip and looked at my boys. After she finished taking pictures, the NICU nurse asked if I wanted to hold them. I finally gave in. That was the best moment of peace in my life... holding my baby boys WAS Heaven on earth. I am glad that I had the chance to hold them. It was my one and only chance to feel the realness of the whole situation. I didn't want to put them down, or say goodbye to them. I wanted them to wake up so badly.

The nurse made a "scrapbook" full of pictures for me. She was so nice. We received two bags, filled with stuff used on the twins, like blankets, measuring tape, and same-sized diapers. There were some clothes, made "with love". In the card were two heart charms, which I wear around my neck.

I gave birth on my husband's birthday, and buried my boys on my grandmother's birthday, in August 2007. We lost them at 22 weeks gestation. With so much going on, I didn't even realize how far along I was. They were two weeks shy of being viable. So did they even try to save them? A week or so later, I saw on TV that some doctors had saved a baby girl born at 22 weeks. Why couldn't they save mine?

After that, the doctor in Houston stopped returning my phone calls. To me, it felt like they were saying, "Well our experiment is over, so we're done". I felt used and hurt. My local OB was very rude to me, too. I refused to go on birth control, and he criticized me for it. To this day, we feel that if that doctor had actually cared, we could have saved the boys.

CHRISTMAN-SCHARER: At the OB, everything was fine. I did not have preeclampsia. The heartbeats were strong. I was 22 weeks, 3 days at this time.

I went back to CHOP at 22 weeks, 5 days. The girls were doing well, although Twin A only had 1cm of fluid while Twin B had 10cm. Since I now officially had TTTS, I had a Level II ultrasound. I was in a lot of pain from all the fluid retention. My right side hurt really badly from the ligaments pulling. I was very uncomfortable.

MORGAN: During a routine ultrasound, they noticed Jadon's foot looked clubbed due to the TTTS. I was informed about treatments for clubbed feet, in case he was born with a deformity. (This never was the case!)

REBILAS: Donor was 378 grams and recipient was 637 grams. We were told we would need to see a specialist almost two hours away. He specialized in the laser surgery we had heard so much about. Our first visit was to do all of the background paperwork. They did the scans on the babies and saw that our donor still had a bladder, which was a good thing. They checked the blood flow from the umbilical cords. They were a little nervous about our donor; his connection to the placenta was on the far side, while our recipient's was in the middle. The recipient was doing well and had no heart issues. They performed my first amnio reduction, taking out 1.5 liters of fluid.

JELLEY: 22 weeks along and again another great appointment: babies all looking good. We had an appointment with a specialist for baby A's heart, because the outer wall had thickened (like every muscle, when worked, it gets larger). Overall, the babies looked perfect. They were all growing at the same pace, and the fluid was pretty close to the same, although I did notice it seemed kind of low. The units were all in the fours and fives. I remember asking if the babies could switch roles, because I noticed that baby C had more fluid than baby A. The doctor said they could, on rare occasions, but this was not a worry in our case. Everything was looking so good, I asked, "So it looks like I could be a laser surgery success story?" The doctor stopped and said, "Well, from what we can see..." I could hear that he was afraid to be too confident, but then again he was always like that.

BENNER: That week came and went; we stayed at a stage 2.

OROSZ: My husband and I went back at 22 weeks to see if there was any improvement from drinking protein shakes. I knew before the doctor came in to go over the ultrasound. I had had so many ultrasounds that I knew what to look for and did my research. I could see that Baby B had no visible bladder and that Baby A had so much more fluid. Of course the tech couldn't tell me anything until the doctor was present, but I remember my OB asking the tech, "Is it?", and she said, "yes". Instantly I burst into tears; it was confirmed. Baby B had no measurable fluid and no visible bladder. Baby A was swimming in a lot of fluid. We were at Stage 2.

My fundal height was at 30, so my doctor recommended us to CHOP and we went there the next day. It was a 5 hour drive from our home, and our son. We had the evaluations: still in Stage 2. Baby A's heart was showing signs of thickening. We were scheduled for laser surgery at 22 weeks, 4 days. Dr. B., who did our surgery, told me the risk of losing one or both. I was a nervous wreck and constantly in tears because I feared losing my boys. As well as the laser surgery, we had amnio reduction. They removed 2 liters of fluid from Baby A. After surgery, they did an ultrasound and we still had two heart-beats! We were overjoyed at that, but didn't get our hopes up. We scheduled a follow up appointment for the next week, to make sure everything had worked and our boys were still alive, but they didn't want to release me to drive the five hours back home, in case something happened. I spent the longest week of my life in the most uncomfortable hotel bed. We went back to CHOP, and our boys were still alive!

FLETCHER: This ultrasound was at 22 weeks 1day. Ab-bigail is on top and Allyson is on the bottom. You can tell the size differ-ence at that time. You can tell how much more Allyson is formed than Ab-bigail. Abbigail's bladder never showed up, which is a sign of TTTS.

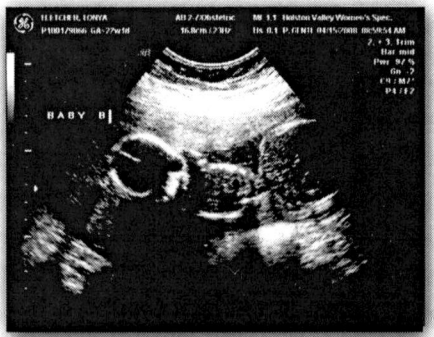
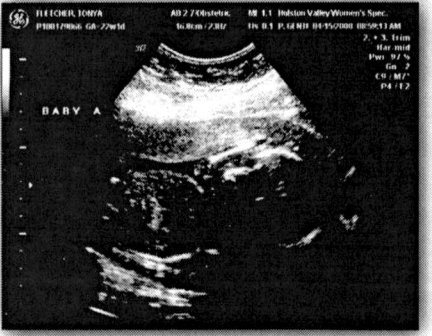

DOBBS: September 22, 2005. Went in for my regular appointment and Dr. P. said I still needed to take it easy. He said he likes all of his twin pregnancies to go to 34 weeks, 36 weeks if possible.

DILLE: We had another ultrasound this week. Cara's condition had improved; her edema was better and her fluid levels were still increasing. Her Dopplers were all normal and there was still no sign of hy-drops. We were beginning to feel better about Cara's chances of survival.

BRUCE: On July 24, 2004 (at 22 weeks 2 days gesta-tion), we went for an ultrasound with the Maternal Fetal Medicine doctor. The twins appeared to be sta-ble. The doctor didn't go into detail about their status. Jordyn weighed 11 ounces, with 2.7cm of fluid in her sac, and Taylor weighed 1.3pounds, with 7.0cm of fluid in her sac. There was a 47% discord between the twins.

17
Week 23

BRUCH: The doctors recommended another amnio reduction. They took another two liters, bringing the grand total to eight liters. The recipient twin was sleeping, so the pain wasn't too bad. It hurt, but nothing like last time. On the TTTS scale, we were now a 3. After the reduction, the doctor admitted me to the hospital. I expected to be hospitalized at 24 weeks, so that wasn't a shocker to me. If we could hold off delivery for one more week, our recipient twin (the larger one) would have a shot at a possible life. The smaller baby (the donor) would need another three to four weeks. To be honest, I didn't think we could keep going at this rate for that amount of time. This was the last day we could do a selection; my husband kept telling me, "We are here for two babies," and to be completely honest, I never thought I could lose both.

HADDIGAN: My OB said I could go back to work part-time.

SLICHTER: On February 15, 2006 I went back to UNC. The trip to this appointment was grim. We were numb. I met with the doctor and had a pelvic exam. The doctor found that I was dilated. He said that my body most likely sensed that something was wrong, and I was going into preterm labor. He also said that I would have delivered naturally in one or two weeks. We decided to go ahead with the termination, and were given the choice of a D and C or a saline abortion. I desperately wanted to see my babies, and couldn't stand the way they perform the D and C, so we chose saline, then went back to the hotel. We were lucky; we had the support of my mother and sister, who quickly drove the 24 hours to be there with us. Without them, I don't think I could have made it through this.

The next day, we went in and waited a few hours for a room to open up. As soon as it did, I got settled and had an extremely large needle inserted into my abdomen. The saline was injected, and in about an hour, my baby fell fast asleep. I was given Pitocin to induce labor, and the next morning I delivered my twins. Since Jack had passed a month before, he was very small and brown and his arms and legs looked like strings; he didn't look like a baby at all. Jake looked like a perfect baby, but he was very small. His underdeveloped skin was bruised from the contractions. We got to spend eight hours with our lifeless babies. I got to take many pictures, and I was just thankful for the time I got to spend with them. The doctors were all very nice and comforting, and did their very best to help me in whatever way that they could. Then we went home, and it was time for the grieving process.

DICK: Around 11:30pm on May 26, 2007, at 23 weeks and 1 day, I woke to a soaking wet bed. Thinking I had peed on myself, I went to the restroom. However, when I got done, I couldn't stop going. "My water broke", I kept thinking over and over. "What now?"

I went and told my husband. He said I had probably peed on myself, but then another gush came. "Oh no, we have to get you to the hospital," he said. We called the hospital and they said to come on in. I went, and after an inspection of my cervix, the doctor said, "Your twins have TTTS; there's nothing we can do about it. Maybe, if they were at least a pound, we could try, but they don't even weigh that. I'm sorry, but you had better be prepared for your girls to die. One of your amniotic sacs has already burst, so it's just a matter of time before you deliver."

I was shocked. "How dare he come in here and tell me he isn't going to do anything for my girls!" I shouted at my husband, "I want to go to an-other hospital!" I couldn't believe that someone who handles this kind of thing on a daily basis could be so heartless to someone in my position. I just wanted to leave. My family talked me into staying, however, considering I was already in labor. I listened to my family and stayed.

On May 29, 2007, I woke around 2 am in the hospital bed, once again soaking wet. This time my other water had broken. I cleaned up and spent the rest of the morning sedated. I started going into labor at exactly 7pm that night. At 7:06 pm, Brookelynn Cheyenne was born into this world, sleeping. She had passed away May 28, 2007 and I hadn't been told. She weighed 1lb. 4oz. Her sister, Jazmen Rene, was born at 7:16pm. She was born into this world alive, and taken after only 15 minutes, at 7:31 pm. She weighed precisely one pound.

TUMMERS: This is where life got interesting. Al-though I still hadn't gained much weight (total gain was at 8 lbs. now), I felt HUGE and was very uncom-fortable. I understood why working only until 28 weeks was important. I'd never find my feet after that!

Geoff and I met with our OB and once again learned that our babies weren't cooperating with him determining their sex. He asked when my next big scan was, and told me it was good that it was that same day. Perhaps this was his way of telling me he saw something that needed further investigation.

The ultrasound that afternoon was actually cancelled by the hospital, but I was stubborn and insisted that they do it anyway since I was there. Thank goodness for my stubborn nature, because it was during that ultrasound that it became obvious something was wrong. After seeing three different people, I was left in the scan room for so they could "check to make sure they had everything". After waiting for 20 minutes, I began to suspect something wasn't right. As soon as my doctor came into the room, I knew, and burst into tears. He tried to reassure me that all was well, but the speed with which I was being sent to the specialist told me that this was very serious. I remember struggling to walk out of the hospital to call my husband, my mom, and our babysitter. I was a mess and very hard to understand. I was so very scared for my babies. I made it five minutes outside the city when my phone rang. It was the doctor, saying I needed to remain calm, but that I must return to the hospital immediately; I was being sent to Toronto, right away. I was to have Geoff come, too, and to meet him on the delivery floor. And then I really wept. I could hardly talk when I called Geoff and our babysitter. It all seemed so unreal.

Reality didn't hit until I got to the hospital and spoke to Dr. H. He explained that he'd spoken to doctors in London, who told him to contact Mt. Sinai in Toronto. The specialist there, after hearing the results of the ultrasound, said it was imperative that we come to Toronto right away. Dr. H. told me I would likely have surgery, and be in Toronto for a week or so. Then he really scared me, telling me I would be given a shot of celesdone, a steroid, to strengthen premature babies' lungs. I cried and shook; my heart was breaking and my mind raced with thoughts of these babies, and the life I wanted for them. How could this be happening to me, to them, to our family?

We arrived in Toronto about 8:30 that night, and were admitted. We had another ultrasound at about 9:00. That was when we found out that the babies were boys, and confirmed that they had twin to twin transfusion syndrome. Everything in our world came to a screeching halt. It was explained to us that one of our sons was transferring fluid to the other. This "donor" twin had no visible bladder and was stuck, with no amniotic fluid around him. The other twin, the "recipient", seemed to be more affected. His cord showed some reverse blood flow, and there was thickening in his heart. He had pockets of 8cm of fluid around him -- the minimum needed to be considered TTTS. Normally in TTTS, the donor baby is smaller than the recipient, but our boys appeared to be about the same size. Our recipient might have been an ounce smaller, actually. This assured the medical staff that our TTTS had only been occurring for a few days. The other discovery was that one baby's cord was inserted very poorly, 11cm away from the placental wall. If we did nothing, there was a 100% chance we would lose at least one baby. Amniotic reduction was not really an option at this stage of the disease. We could have the laser surgery performed there, at Mt. Sinai, the only place it was done

in Canada. It came with risks, though, including pre-
term labor. If that happened, we would lose both babies, as they were too small to be viable.

　　We left the scan feeling scared, but confident
that they would save our babies and correct the problem. The hospital brought in a cot in for my husband,
and gave us a private room. We sat together and
cried and prayed and talked. We were so scared, but
both of us tried to be strong. We talked about names
for our boys, and decided on Cameron and Cole.
Geoff suggested that maybe one of the boys should be
named after the man who was about to perform life-
saving surgery for them, the head of fetal medicine,
Dr. R.

　　The next morning, we met Dr. R.; we were
amazed by his gentle nature and knew we were in
great hands. We were warned that Cole was a sick
baby, but nothing seemed real to us. As scared as we
were, negative thoughts didn't cross our minds. Our
focus was on our wonderful boys and all the fun we
would have with them. The ultrasound he then performed showed that the reverse cord flow had increased in frequency, and the fluid pocket around
Cole was up to 10cm. Surgery was scheduled for as
soon as possible. Discussion turned to the best place
to enter the uterus, which seemed to take a long time.
I had an anterior placenta, and what I now know was
a velamentous cord insertion on our recipient, though
none of those terms were given to us. We did hear
terms like "acute TTTS", but had no idea what that
meant.

　　The surgery took place at 5:00 that afternoon.
Dr. R. spoke to us after the surgery and told us that he

was very confident that he had gotten all of the affected vessels, and that there were quite a number of them. The most serious ones were located where the membrane attached to the placenta, and a septostomy had been necessary in order to get to them. This, in essence, meant that our boys were now mono mono twins, which meant frequent ultrasounds, and probably hospitalization after 28 weeks. When the hole was created, my husband later shared with me, our donor baby reached through it to his very sick twin, like he was reaching out to reassure him. Dr. R. went on to tell us that when he checked the boys at the start of the surgery, the fluid pockets had increased again. Cole's abdomen was now completely full of fluid, which meant our TTTS was at Stage 4. His heart was also much worse than before. Because of this, Dr. R. sent me for a fetal echocardiogram the following morning.

The day started out great. I felt strong movements and we had a good feeling about the fetal echocardiogram. We were excited to find out how our boys were doing, expecting to hear from the doctor that both of the boys were going to be keeping me uncomfortable for the next thirteen weeks.

Then, our world came to a sudden and frightening halt. The words "This baby has no heartbeat. Your baby has died. I'm sorry, your baby passed away," will be forever etched in my brain. We were completely blown away, devastated. Yet I was still expected to lie quietly while the cardiologist checked our surviving twin. My husband had to leave the room, and I was alone, except for this doctor, who seemed heartless.

When Geoff returned, the cardiologist told us that all seemed fine with the other baby. We asked what this meant for the survivor. He said everything should be fine, but that Dr. R. would confirm that.

What about the other baby? What will happen now? These were my questions. The most devastating (and incorrect) answer was given to me: "Your body will just absorb him." I sobbed and sobbed. Not only was I not going to have my twins together, and not only was I now the mother of an angel baby, but I was never going to meet my angel. It would be like my baby never existed. We were quietly left alone in the heart clinic while the doctor called for a porter, and let the floor nurses know what had happened. We held each other and sobbed. Geoff had a very tough time remaining still, and kept leaving me to go make calls telling our family and close friends.

Dr. R. came after the staff called and told him what had happened. He scanned me again and confirmed that Cole's heart had been very, very sick and he'd gone into heart failure. His abdomen was even more full of fluid now, in death, than it had been the night before. Our concern now was Cameron, as his MCA (middle cerebral artery) readings showed anemia and ascites (fluid around his abdomen). Dr. R. was very confident that all vessels had been cauterized, and that this change was due to a final rush of fluid from Cameron to Cole as the last vessels were sealed. Much scanning and rescanning was done, to see if the MCA was high enough to warrant a blood transfusion -- another risky procedure. However, this wasn't all they were looking at. One doctor devastatingly told us they needed to make sure that a blood transfusion wasn't pointless, just saving a very sick baby. Eventually, it was determined that it needed to be done, very soon, and the transfusion was scheduled for as soon as the blood was available.

My parents arrived and we were all very emotional. My parents had been so very overjoyed about us having twins. My mom had shopped her heart out just weeks before, buying two of everything (well, actually three, since my brother and his wife were also expecting). My dad is a fairly emotional guy when it comes to us kids, especially his only daughter. It was a very tough afternoon and evening, waiting for the blood to be ready.

My dad stayed with me for the procedure, which was very touching and very comforting. The room was filled with staff: three doctors, two nurses assisting Dr. R., a nurse helping with the blood transfusion and a lab technician. The procedure was a bit uncomfortable, as they used a needle similar to an amnio needle and put it in at two or three different places. They removed a sample of blood and checked the hemoglobin levels right there in the procedure room. Cameron was given 40 cc's of blood. After cleaning me up, I was wheeled back to my room to wait and hope and pray that my remaining twin would indeed survive, and that there would be no damage to his brain.

The next day, they checked his MCA and, thankfully, it was already coming down. They then checked my cervix, which was closed and long, and sent me home with a follow-up and MRI's scheduled for later that week. That drive home was one of the strangest I think I will ever have; it seemed to take forever, and yet it was like we had never left Monkton. I will never forget that eerie feeling. As we drove into town, we both cried as we realized how completely and eternally different our lives were now than when we left for work only three days before.

CHRISTMAN-SCHARER: I went back to CHOP at 23 weeks, 3 days, and had a fetal echocardiogram and ultrasound. We talked about laser surgery and amnio reduction. Twin B (Kylie) had thickening around her heart due to TTTS. We decided not to do the laser surgery due to my placental issues.

When I was 23 weeks, 4 days, I went back to the perinatologists for my first amnio reduction. They took 2 liters (wow) of fluid out of Kylie's sack. The pain in my side disappeared once they removed that fluid, and boy did my belly shrink. I had looked about 7 – 8 months pregnant before. Afterwards, I looked like I should. Twin A (Karlyn) had a little over 1 cm of fluid and Twin B (Kylie) had 11 cm. I had contractions for an hour after the procedure. Later, we went to the NICU for an early tour, since they knew we were going to be delivering early.

I also had an appointment with my ob-gyn, at 23 weeks, 7 days. The girls sounded good and everything was progressing ok.

REBILAS: When we arrived at our appointment with the specialist, they started with another amnio reduction. This time, they removed a liter of fluid from our recipient. We were given options for our babies. We were told that we could do one of three things: abort and start over because we were young, do a cord coagulation and tie off one baby to save the other, or do nothing and risk both their lives. We were already emotionally drained by this point and did not like any of our options. We wanted to fix it! We told them the abortion was not an option for us at all. We would go and home and think and pray on it. They urged us to do the ligation, saying it was the only chance at having at least one baby. We wrestled with this, thinking, "Could we really just give up on our donor baby like that?" What made up our minds entirely entirely was being informed that they would be taking the recipient, because he was "easier to get to". That didn't make any sense to us. They were also urging us to travel across states to see a doctor within three days, because he was going on vacation. It all sat wrong with us. We decided, then and there, that we would do what we could, but we were leaving it up to the Lord! For His Glory, we would live with the outcome.

BENNER: I regret now never going on bed rest. I did ask, every visit, if I should, but the doctor told me it wouldn't really help. I should have done it anyway, but I didn't, and I regret that every day. Maybe, just maybe, I could have changed the outcome. But I must not do that, because it is an awful thing to wonder about the "WHAT IFS".

At 23 weeks, we took serious action. Along with Dr. R., we decided the laser surgery might be the best thing; we had tried everything and the boys seemed fine, but weren't. They kicked daily, like crazy. We got in touch with Dr. L. at UCSF in San Francisco. He told us we would have an 85% chance of one surviving and a 50% chance for both. He also said I was a great candidate for the surgery. His words were kind, and gave us hope.

A day after making our decision, we had plane tickets. We had prayed and prayed so much, but it ended up that everything was turning for the worse. We had so much hope and faith. Every week, when we went to the doctor, we never knew if the babies were going to be alive. That was awful.

On the day of my appointment at UCSF, we went to the ultrasound and tests. I was in a little pain, but nothing totally unusual. I didn't let it get to me; I was trying to save my babies. They took forever to do the ultrasound and I was mad, uncomfortable and pregnant! They did a vaginal ultrasound, and said my cervix was short. The next thing I knew, I was being rushed to OB and maternity. I had THREE doctors in my room all at once. They said the babies were not going to make it. I was in preterm labor and there was nothing they could do. They feared that all three of us wouldn't last, that I would develop preeclampsia. I knew everything wasn't okay when Jacob broke down. My body was ready, the babies were ready, but they had no chance of surviving at 23weeks 4days. We couldn't make it a few weeks more. I was dilated, but the babies were kicking as if nothing was wrong. I couldn't stop crying. Jacob, my mom, and I were all devastated. I tried everything to keep them here, alive and inside, as long as possible.

The NICU doctor came down to talk to us; if Isiah came out alive, it would be a matter of minutes before he passed. "Multiples sometimes don't make it, even at 24 weeks. Everything is worse when you have multiples," was all that he told us. He suggested I go to our hotel, because it wasn't right for me to lie there listening to all the babies crying, and other mothers in labor. I couldn't sleep that night as my contractions got stronger and I was in pain. I woke my husband and mom, and said, "I need to go to the hospital. I can't take it anymore."

At 5 am, I was given an IV and fluids. I was dilated to a 3. Pitocin was started at 7am and my water broke at around noon, on its own. I couldn't make up my mind about an epidural, so I received fentanyl, and 11 hours later had the urge to push. Mason Andrew, 1LB 9.2oz, came at 11:36pm, and Isiah Caleb, 1LB 0.2oz, at 11:46. They were so tiny, didn't cry, didn't open their eyes, and were so beautiful. They had Jacob's nose, my lips and ears, and long legs. They were given morphine to keep them at peace. Mason passed about an hour later and Isiah at three. I knew he was a fighter. The one thing I wanted was to hold them.

WRIGHT: I was brought in one last time before the 24 week mark, so that the doctors could try to convince me once more to terminate my pregnancy. When we refused two of the doctors, they sent in the head of the entire Maternal-Fetal Medicine Group. He told us that this was not the baby we wanted and we needed to abort. We were determined to give our little girl every chance at survival and refused them once again.

BRAY: On Friday, the 20th of March, 2009, Dr. D. confirmed TTTS. He told us that we were in stage 3 of the disease, and that had we had been left untreated another week, both twins would have died. The ultrasound showed Oligohydraminos in the donor sac; no bladder was visible. Polyhydraminos was found in the recipient's sac, and an enlarged bladder. Dr. D. explained the Dopplers he had taken of the umbilical cord. The diastolic flow was absent in the donor twin and reversed in the recipient twin. Our babies were very sick. Dr. D. went over our options, explaining that if we did not have the laser treatment, there was a very high chance we would lose both our babies. There was no other option, in my eyes. I would do all I could to save my babies.

We had the laser treatment that day; the procedure was not at all painful. I had a lot of sedation, and Dr. D. was very calming. They drained two liters of fluid from my recipient's sac. The pain in my back went away and I instantly felt much more comfortable. Dr. D. was very pleased with the surgery. After the treatment, I was sent home and told to rest. I would go back to the hospital on the following Monday, for a follow up scan. We were warned that there was a high risk of premature labor, so I must rest as much as possible. That weekend went so slow; all Gareth and I could do was pray.

The day finally came, and the scan showed good news -- the treatment seemed to have worked. Our donor baby (Oliver) was producing fluid, and a bladder was now visible. Our recipient baby (Thomas) was now producing less fluid and showed signs of improvement. We were so happy and thankful for all the staff at St. Michael's. However, our babies were not out of the woods. Oliver's sac had a small tear, and was leaking amniotic fluid. Dr. D. explained that this meant a high risk of miscarriage. We had another scan with Dr. D.; he was pleased with the twins' progress and happy to let local hospital take over our care. I had weekly scans at Royal Glamorgan Hospital (RGH) and everything seemed stable. I started to relax slightly, and began enjoying my pregnancy again.

That is, until one Saturday morning, when Gareth was at work and I was at home with William. I stood up to get myself a drink, and pop - I felt my water break! The first feeling I had was panic! This could not be happening; I was only 23 weeks and 1 day gestation. My babies were too small to be born! I grabbed the telephone and headed straight for the bathroom. I phoned the hospital and they told me to get there as soon as possible. I got in touch with Gareth and we headed to the hospital right away. The trip took forever. I sobbed and sobbed. There was nothing I could do but pray!

When we finally arrived at the hospital, I was taken to a room where they placed a monitor on me. "I have found both heartbeats," the midwife reassured me, "Your babies are ok at the moment." She asked me how many weeks along I was. We then had to sit and wait for a doctor to come to scan the twins. He confirmed that our donor twin's membranes had ruptured! Then, he sat next to me and asked how I was feeling. I started crying again. He explained that 23 weeks gestation was "very cloudy", and he "tends to go with the parents' choice at this point". He said, "Children born at this gestation have been known to survive, but there is a very good chance that both babies will die. 23 weeks is very premature; if your babies were to survive, the risk of disability would be extremely high." That didn't matter to us. I understood all the risks, but to me, there was no other option. I wanted my babies to have the best possible care, and the best possible chance at life.

We were told that if we chose to give my babies active care, we would have to be admitted to a hospital that had a neo natal unit appropriate for babies as premature as ours. I was transferred via ambulance to South Mead Hospital in Bristol.

OROSZ: I was on bed rest for weeks 24 to 26, and had weekly ultrasounds at my doctor after returning from Philadelphia. We were lucky that my husband's work was supportive, letting him work steady daylight; usually he worked swing shifts. My mom and gram came over during the day, while he was at work. They helped me with my house work and my son. I was not to lift anything.

WALLINGTON: I continued to be on bed rest, but at 23 weeks, another problem occurred. At a regular appointment with my OB, while checking my cervix length, they realized I was beginning to funnel and needed to be hospitalized immediately. I was scheduled to have a cerclage put in the next day, and remained in the hospital for ten days, on magnesium sulfate to stop my contractions. When I was released, I was to stay in bed as much as possible, and was prescribed medicine to take every 4 hours to prevent contractions. By this time, you can only imagine the fear and simple exhaustion within me. I knew that I had to be strong for my girls. I knew I was their number one chance. I tried not to think of the "what ifs", and kept my heart in the Lord. I was not sure of what the outcome would be, but I knew it was His plan, and that I could only do what I could control.

JELLEY: I went to see the heart specialist, thinking something wasn't right. The babies' movement had decreased a lot, and I kept thinking about what I would do if I found out one or more of my babies were gone. I told myself to stop worrying, but it was like waiting for the other shoe to drop. I went to the appointment and everything looked fine. The doctor was just looking at the babies' hearts, but since I asked, he checked that all three hearts were beating.

18
Week 24

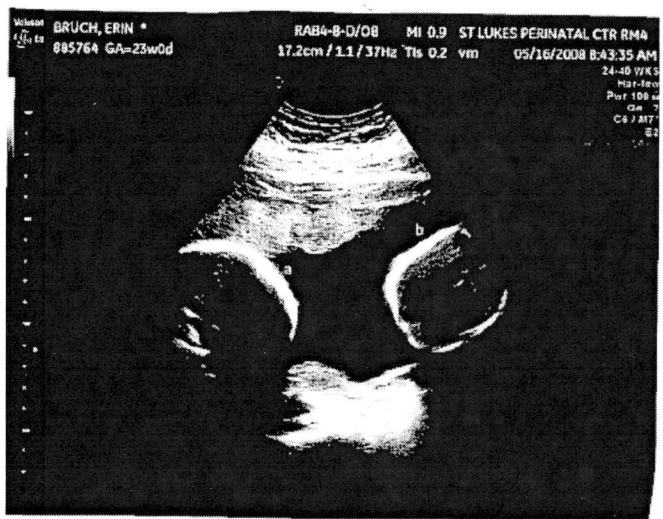

BRUCH: We had an ultrasound early that first full day in the hospital. We could see a reverse flow of blood in the recipient's cord. We could either deliver them then, or let the recipient die and hope that the donor survived. We chose to deliver. The doctors used less pain medication during the c-section, so the babies would be awake for the NICU staff. Halfway through the c-section, after the boys were out, I regained feeling and felt them sewing me up. It was so painful. When the anesthesiologist and doctors realized what had happened, they freaked out a bit. I remember one yelling, "Get me 2 doses of morphine…" Then, after what seemed like hours, the same doctor yelled, "Fentanyl! Get me a dose of fentanyl, STAT!"

Happily, at 3:24 pm both of our boys were born by a classic c-section. The recipient baby, Thomas Matthew Bruch (1 lb. 3oz., 11.5 inches long), cried when he was born. The donor baby, Vincent Sterling Bruch, was 11oz., and 10.25 inches long. We were only 24 weeks along, and they were already born. I now had to put my faith in the NICU team, and wait. The twins were here, and I was still helpless. A nurse commented on how small they were, and the doctor told her to be quiet. It was horrible to hear her say that, even though it was true.

HADDIGAN: Week 24 - Bleeding and lots of it! The OB nurse said to stay in bed over the weekend and to call if anything else happened. Two days later I woke in the middle of the night with CONTRACTIONS! We went to the hospital, where I was admitted. The placenta was separating and I would need to stay there, on strict bed rest. Being in the hospital was the worst! Not just because it's boring and the food is awful, but because being away from family and friends, all alone, worrying about what would happen next, was terrible. Every day was filled with doctors and nurses, all telling me something different, but all saying that the babies were doing fine, and that the longer they were in there, the better off they would be.

TUMMERS: Three days after we left, we returned to Toronto to have a fetal MRI. It was a horrible experience, but thankfully, fairly short (compared to what they had prepared me for). Two days after that, we returned again to meet with Dr. R.'s team at the Special Pregnancy Program clinic. I did the formal intake interview, which would normally occur BEFORE surgery, at time of diagnosis -- another realization of just how critical our situation had been. I was scanned briefly, and breathed a huge sigh of relief when I saw Cameron's heart beating. Then, back out to the waiting room, until the nurse who did the thorough scan was ready for us.

We requested a meeting with a social worker; we had yet to meet with anyone to discuss our loss, or its implications. No one from the hospital had offered this service the weekend before, which shocked us. The social worker was pleasant, though I didn't feel a real connection with her. We also had a surprise visit from the doctor that did our intake assessment. She expressed her sympathy to us, and then was blunt: this was not the outcome she expected at our first scan, not at all what things had looked like at that point.

Then the nurse did the full scan. She showed us the results for his MCA, just above the 95th percentile. This worried us, but everything else seemed fine. His growth was great, almost 600 grams, which was a huge gain. He now had fluid and a bladder. Dr. R. came in and scanned me as well. He got much better MCA readings and told us that everything was now in the normal range. Finally, we had received news to feel joy about.

CHRISTMAN-SCHARER: I had another appointment with perinatologists, and a level 1 ultrasound. Baby A (Karlyn) was a little anemic and Baby B (Kylie) still had thickening of the heart. Baby A had 1.62 cm of fluid and Baby B had 14 cm. The amnio reduction hadn't worked. I got a steroid shot to help the lungs grow, so that if they were born early, they would have a chance. Though we wanted it to go longer, our goal at that point was delivery at 28 weeks, when the girls would have a better chance of survival. My cervix was fine, but they were watching for preterm labor.

The night I went back for my second steroid shot, I had a scare. I had really bad low back pain, from my legs to my upper belly. I was sent to the hospital to get checked out. There, they said it was pressure on my nerves, from all the fluid retention. They also found a bacterial infection, so they gave me an antibiotic. The babies were moving a lot. I loved to feel them move. It put me in a peaceful state.

MORGAN: During a routine ultrasound, they saw a white mark on Jadon's heart and said it's a sign of Downs Syndrome. Once again, I broke down in tears on the drive home. (This was never the case, either.)

REBILAS: We spoke with Dr. Q's office and were told that I was 'probably too heavy' to have the surgery, that it wasn't worth the trip. (I was 23 weeks pregnant with twins and weighed 225 pounds.)

We traveled to see Dr. D. and scheduled the laser surgery. He was amazing! When we arrived, we found him waiting for us in the garage with a wheel chair. He personally wheeled me inside, placed my IV, and took me for the ultrasound. He was so caring and compassionate that we knew this was where we were supposed to be! After our scans, he felt that our diagnosis wasn't as bad as we were lead to believe. He thought that with continued bed rest and Ensure, we had a good chance to have TWO survivors! He was the first doctor to say it and believe it!

JELLEY: My sisters kept asking if more people could come to my ultrasound: my nieces, and a friend that hadn't seen an ultrasound before. I told them that I wasn't sure; every appointment was filled with worry that something was wrong, which wouldn't be fun. I ended up saying that it was ok, though, as long as they stayed in the waiting room until we determined that everything was ok.

I told the ultrasound tech that I felt very little movement. In fact, I had noticed no movement on the right side, which was where babies A and C were. She said, "Let's take a look and set your mind at ease." The worst moment in the world was when she started to check and there was no movement. I had had so many ultrasounds that I knew almost exactly what I was looking at, and nothing looked right. The tech started to figure out which baby was where, and traced where they were. Everything in me screamed, "I know where my babies are, I just need to see heartbeats!" but I asked only, "See heartbeats?" I knew she normally would not tell me herself and would wait for the doctor, but I suspect she recognized that I knew what I was looking at. She said, "Well, I see one for sure," way too calmly.

When she went to get the doctor, I asked my sister for my phone. She started to say, "Just wait. I don't think she thought it was final yet." My voice broke, but I don't think I was crying yet. I said, "No, I need my phone." I called Cody but he didn't answer, so I texted CALL ME NOW. He called seconds later. No one should ever have to tell their husband that two of his children have gone to heaven. The emotions are flooding me as I write this. I hung up to hear what the doctor was saying; it was like a terrible dream. I didn't really cry yet.

The doctor said yes, the babies were "demised". I hate that word; it kind of sounds evil. He went on to say that baby A had no fluid, and baby C had a lot as well as hydrops. Baby A was too curled

up in a ball from lack of fluid to see if she did, also.
He went on to look at the survivor, baby B, and it
didn't look good. Her heart was under stress and her
fluid was extremely low. After the tech measured
baby B, the doctor said he would admit me to the
hospital, where I would discuss with the neonatologist the odds of her living if delivered at 24 weeks.
He also repeated that some people chose to let nature
do its thing and not interfere. I don't think he was
trying to push this, but rather, felt I needed to know
the option. It helped that he said, "I think I know
what you are going to choose." He knew I didn't believe in selective reduction.

I called Cody back. I started to tell him that
baby B was in trouble and needed to be monitored, he
interrupted me, "What about the other two?" (I had
told him in our earlier phone call.) It was then that I
started to really cry. I said they were gone, and I
know he broke down, too. We spent a little time crying over the phone, before Cody said he would look
into coming home right away.

My sister took me to the hospital, all the while
trying to talk about random things. She said I needed
to consider whether my baby would have a good
quality of life, if she were delivered at 24 weeks. I
tried to say, firmly, "I'm not thinking about it." I
didn't add what I was thinking: I already lost two; I'm
NOT going to choose to lose my only survivor.

I honestly didn't care what the neonatologist
told me. She put together a formula that said my
baby had a 59% chance of survival, and didn't ac-
count for any disabilities she may have. She said, "So,
you and your husband need to discuss what you

want to do." I said, "Actually, I'm very confident my husband and I agree. We are going to do everything possible to save our baby." My doctor came in, and asked if we were getting aggressive. I said YES. So they gave me a steroid shot and magnesium for her brain. That night was very emotional and scary. I didn't sleep at all. Cody was able to call and text because he was in a different time zone, two hours later than me, and they got him up at 2 in the morning for training.

I was having trouble breathing and my pulse was 120 -130 when they started talking about my many risk factors for getting a form of hydrops myself, where my lungs would fill with fluid. But test after test came back normal, so they decided that it wasn't anything. My baby's heartbeat didn't decelerate as badly when they put me on oxygen, so they questioned whether the lack of oxygen had affected my babies.

The next morning, Betty, the same ultrasound tech I had seen each time, did a scan of baby B. Though she was only checking baby B, I kept seeing my other babies... still there, not moving. Afterwards, I went into the bathroom and lost it. When I came out, the nurse asked if I was ok. "You just kept coughing. Sounded pretty bad." She commented. I guess no one realized how broken my heart was... is.

Cody got home the next afternoon. It felt so weird to be so sad, yet so excited to see him after so long. Baby B did great all weekend. The nurse kept saying that she liked her daddy, because whenever he was close, her heart rate was where it was supposed to be. We had a lot of breakdowns that weekend. I missed my girls' movement. Although I wanted baby B to wait, I really wanted the others to come out before they were messed up any more. I would sit there and tell them how sorry I was that I couldn't do anything. Cody had to go back on Monday. Letting him go was so scary, but we were assured he would graduate early and be back by the end of the week.

BRAY: I was admitted to the hospital, and bed rest was not fun. I wondered how long I would be there, and found out that I needed to get to 28 weeks.

DOBBS: On October 6, 2005, we went to see Dr. P. for another ultrasound. Things looked good; he wanted me to start coming once a week, and to take it easy.

BRUCE: On August 6, 2007, my Mother-in-Law and I went to see my Maternal Fetal Medicine doctor for an ultrasound. I was at 24 weeks 1 day. Jordyn weighed 15 oz. and Taylor weighed 1.11 lbs., which was a 48% discord. Taylor was doing well, actually growing on track, and the fluid in her sac measured 8.8 cm. Jordyn, on the other hand, was not doing so well. She had only 2.2 cm of fluid in her sac, and the hydrocephalus had grown worse.

During my discussion with the doctor, he noticed that I was writing down notes on a pad that I had brought to the appointment. He asked me if I was making a "scrapbook." I was actually writing down the answers to all the questions the TTTS specialist had told me to ask. At this comment, I realized that I wanted another Maternal Fetal Medicine doctor. But, could I get one at 24 weeks? I decided to stick it out with this doctor. I was already in fear of losing my girls at any moment; I didn't think I could add the stress of finding another doctor to my load.

19
Week 25

TUMMERS: I had a regular OB visit this week. It felt unreal to walk into the hospital where it all began. I went over to the nurse, to ask if I needed to keep my pre-admit appointment 10 days later, since there was little chance I would be able to deliver in that hospital. I began to cry. She took me to a private room and had the doctor come in right away. Dr. H. came in, took my hand, and said, "I am so sorry. This was so not how I thought this was going to end."

We discussed my care, and the referral he needed to make to the high risk specialist in our area. It was two days before Christmas; it might take a few days to get it all arranged. Until then, I would continue to visit the local clinic once a week, and have scans as often as the high-risk clinic in London wanted.

He scanned me briefly, showing us a few things that had changed in my placenta. It was heart-breaking to see Cole not moving. We began grief counseling with a local social worker that same day. It was good to talk about my feelings, but I felt she was really trying to help our marriage and not our grief.

CHRISTMAN-SCHARER: On Friday, I had another perinatal appointment, at 25 weeks. They did another amnio reduction, removing 3 liters (oh my goodness!) Twin A (Karlyn) had about 1 cm and Twin B (Kylie) had 15 cm of fluid. Afterwards, I had contractions for about an hour. The amnio reductions hurt and left my belly really tender. On my youngest son's birthday, 6/4/06, we just had a small party for family because of everything I was going through with the girls!

The following Monday, I had another appointment with the perinatal group. I was 25 weeks, 4 days. Baby A (Karlyn) had 2.5 cm of fluid; it went up! Baby B (Kylie) had 8.32 cm. They said they could see both girls' bladders, and that everything looked OK so far.

By Wednesday (25 weeks, 6 days), Baby A (Karlyn) had a fluid level of 1.9 cm and Baby B (Kylie) was back up to 10 cm. Karlyn weighed 1 lb., 2 oz. and Kylie was 2 lbs., 2 oz. They said I might need another amnio reduction.

On Thursday, everything looked good. Heartbeats were strong. I had the 3rd amnio reduction. After removing .5 liters of fluid, Baby A had 3.4 cm of fluid, and we did not see her bladder. Baby B had 5 cm of fluid. My cervix was ok.

REBILAS: I spent a week in the hospital due to contractions, and was put on much more strict bed rest. The doctors did a second amnio reduction and took out .5 liters of fluid. Donor was 14 to 16 ounces (kept changing) and the recipient was 1 pound 9 ounces! Recipient was still hydrops free and doing amazingly. Donor was still growing, which was a great thing. He had a visible bladder, but he had an absent end diastolic flow with his cord, which was something to keep an eye on.

While in the hospital, I was given a tour of the NICU. There was a little, 24-week-old girl there that I got to see. I just watched her growing and knew that my boys could do that, too! I just knew we were going to be ok at that point.

BRAY: Another week down! It was a very stressful time for my family and me. Not only was I away from my 2 year old son, but South Mead was a long way from my home in South Wales.

FLETCHER: I saw Doctors L. and B. that week. When we saw Dr. L., Ally and Abby's heartbeats were the same, 145. I thought that was neat. Dr. L. talked about starting steroid shots and then went to see Dr. B. He came in the room and said, "We are going to try to save baby A." He hated saying those words, but he had to tell us. I received the steroid shot. I had a feeling of helplessness, but I had to stay strong for everyone around me.

I saw the two birds again that week, but it was different this time. They flew together, but then one would fly off in the other direction. I thought, "This is a sign from God that one of my babies isn't going to make it." I kept hoping and praying that everything would be ok, but I knew God's Will would be done. I had a God-given peace that everything would be ok, no matter what happened.

DOBBS: More blood work. One of the babies was 1 pound, 14oz. The other was 1 pound. The next few appointments were uneventful, and we began to get the nursery ready.

JELLEY: I waited, praying every day that little tiny baby B would continue to hold her own. On Monday, my baby was 24 weeks 5 days. They did another ultrasound, and although she was still low on fluid, she looked good. But when the doctor checked her heart rate, it was too low. He walked out into the hall, and I became surrounded by nurses. In seconds, they were inserting another IV (mine had come out the day before), and I finally realized they were slowly getting me ready to take her out. Instantly, I was in tears. The doctor asked the nurse to stand, holding the monitor, while he explained that my baby had de-celled for 5 minutes. He said he would allow up to four short decells, but no more of the long ones. I kept praying that my baby would wait for her daddy. Thankfully, she did ok for the rest of the day.

Soon I started having contractions. At first, I thought they were just Braxton Hicks, but then they started to hurt, off and on. It was just so confusing. It hurt so much, and although I had two babies naturally, it was hard to have pain that wasn't getting me anywhere. The doctor didn't even want to check what they were doing, not worried about me going into labor. He said that if I did, he wouldn't try and stop it; I'd just let have the babies naturally. To me, this was good news, because I really didn't want a c-section, though I didn't get my hopes too high. Every time I had a contraction, my baby decelled. However, since they lasted less than a minute, no one was worried yet. I thought if I had regular labor, with long contractions, it would probably be too much.

Every time I asked Cody about the babies' names, he shut down. He said it was just too much. We had discussed three names and Cody said he liked them, but never said, "OK, yes, I want those names." Finally I called him and said I had to name my girls, it was time. He said he liked the names I had picked, so I announced them to everyone: Emmalin Mercy (Baby

A), Ellina Joy (Baby B), and Ellianna Hope (Baby C).
Ellianna means "God has answered", and Hope because we still had some. Ellina means "bright", and I
hoped that she would be my bright joy.

Three days later, at 25 weeks, 1 day, Ellina's
bio-physical profile came back at 6 out of 8 (2 points
off because of low fluid). Then, the doctor found another pocket of fluid; she was actually 8/8. It was
nice to hear the doctor say, "Another good day. Each
day longer is one week less in the NICU."

My contractions continued that day, but the
baby started to handle them better, although she
would move away from the monitor because the ctx
was squeezing her. The nurse came in once, and
asked why I looked so scared. I tried to breathe
through the pain and find the baby. I was so afraid
something would happen to her and then it would be
too late.

We took a tour through the NICU and saw the
tiniest babies. One was born at 13 oz.! It was amazing, and I was a little encouraged at how well those
tiny, tiny babies were doing. Ellina already had an
estimated weight of 1 lb. 6 oz., so she would be plenty
big. I did ok, but got a bit stressed and sad watching
the monitors.

I went into hard labor Thursday night. Cody
was supposed to fly home Friday morning. After the
scariest, worst labor of my life, I gave birth to my little
girls. Ellina was born first and took a breath all on
her own. I was told she cried, but I was so busy having the other two babies that I didn't hear.

BRUCE: On August 15, 2007, at 25 weeks 3 days, we had an ultrasound at the Maternal Fetal Medicine office. This time, a fetal cardiologist was present. Jordyn weighed 1.2 lbs. and Taylor weighed 2.3 lbs. The cardiologist noticed that Taylor's heart was beginning to thicken and wanted to keep a close watch on it.

20
Week 26

TUMMERS: At the start of the week, we saw a different OB for a scan and the usual checks. All seemed
well with Cameron, but he was presenting in the
breech position. We still had not heard from the high
risk clinic, so our OB called and found out their office
was closed. He assured us that they would get it
booked as soon as possible. In the meantime, if anything happened, or if I felt concerned about lack of
movement or anything, I should come right up to the
labor and delivery floor. He was on call, and would
inform the nurses of our situation. Most of all, he assured me that everyone would know one of our babies had passed away; I would not need to give my
history.

Five days later, I awoke in the middle of the
night. When I rolled over, I felt a popping sensation
and a slight wetness. I'd been to the bathroom only
an hour, earlier so I was certain my bladder wasn't
full. I got up and realized I had brown spotting, and
some mild fluid loss. I called the labor and delivery
floor, who told me to come up and get checked out.
They put me in triage, checked me internally, and saw
nothing. As there were no signs, they felt it couldn't
be my water breaking. They had me walk for an hour,
to see if anything else happened, and called the hospital in London to confirm they would accept me if
need be.

After a few hours, they sent me home but said
to come back at 9:00 for an ultrasound, just to be safe.
When we returned home, as soon as I rolled over in

bed again, it was apparent that this was a major fluid loss. We returned, prepared to be admitted to some hospital, somewhere. Unfortunately, it was at that point we learned London had closed their antenatal ward (a very small ward of only 14 beds), and the NICU had no beds. My stress level quickly increased, but thankfully no contractions were apparent. We were transferred by ambulance back to Toronto, which was very reassuring. Initially, Dr. R. and his team were unsure whether this was a full rupture of membranes, as Cameron's fluid levels still looked good, but I was admitted and the antibiotic protocol for pPROM was begun.

CHRISTMAN-SCHARER: At my appointment with the perinatal group, at 26 weeks, 4 days, we could see Baby A's bladder again, and my cervix was ok. Baby A had 3.54 cm of fluid and Baby B had 7.8 cm. Everything was as good as could be with TTTS.

However, at 26 weeks, 6 days, we could not see Baby A's bladder. Her fluid level was 3.5 cm and Baby B's had increased to9.8 cm. Though the babies were doing ok, and their heartbeats were strong, I would need another amnio reduction in 2 days. At my ob-gyn appointment the next day, I was told I had gained a total of 30 lbs. already.

REBILAS: Donor was 1 pound 5 ounces and recipient was 2 pounds 3 ounces! That week, we got to have a 3D ultrasound. It was amazing to see our little boys in the womb, where they were so peaceful while fighting this battle.

DILLE: I woke up New Year's morning having some big contractions. Then all of a sudden, I felt like I needed to push. The feeling didn't go away, so I told my husband to call 911. I was rushed to the hospital with the best NICU. Though the ambulance ride took probably 20 minutes or so, it felt like an hour or two. My husband was not with me; he had to get our other children into the car, and drove behind us. I was so scared that I was going to deliver in the ambulance. Shortly after I arrived at the hospital, the feeling of having to push lessened, so I was monitored for several hours and then sent home. I wasn't having contractions anymore, either, and the doctors weren't sure exactly what had happened, but they thought perhaps one of the girls had been pushed too close to my cervix. I was so relieved that I wasn't in pre-term labor!

BRAY: Another week down!

OROSZ: My doctor took me off of bed rest at 26 weeks. Both babies had improved tremendously by then. I would need bi-weekly scans after 28 weeks, because Baby A (recipient) showed signs of anemia during the Doppler of his brain. My OB said the donor baby is usually the one that ends up with anemia, because of his low fluid, but in our case, it was the recipient.

FLETCHER: This was a week we will never forget. 26 weeks 2 days, a Tuesday. Erin was doing the ultrasound before Dr. L. came in. I was looking at the screen, and thought there was something different about the picture. It looked like there was a shadow over Abby. When Dr. L. did come, he looked at the ultrasound and confirmed our worst fears. Sometime between the last visit with him and this one, Abby had grown her angel wings to fly away to heaven.

We were both in such shock that it took a while for what we had just heard to sink in.

I remember him talking to us about what would happen next. At first it was about getting us to 30 or more weeks, but it turned into getting us just to the next day or week. The longer they were in the womb, the better their chance at survival. Everyone there was so nice throughout it all, so understanding.

As they left the room, we both broke down, only to have to pull ourselves together again to leave the office. We both felt like the world should have stopped. A piece of both of us died that day, a piece that will never be mended until we are with her in heaven one day.

I remember having to tell people. I couldn't even find the words to say that Abby had left us. The hardest thing we have ever had to do was tell our 4 year old son, Austin, that one of his sisters had gone to heaven. It took him a while to understand that she had gone to heaven, but he is an amazing little boy. He is so sweet and loving and a wonderful big brother.

I started having labor pains that week and was admitted to the hospital. I thought that was it, but again, God wasn't done with us just yet. He was in control, and He knew what He was doing. They watched me closely and then sent me home. I was back on Monday.

21
Week 27

HADDIGAN: During week 27, our donor's heart rate started sounding odd. There was an inconsistency in the rhythm. They were doing non-stress tests and finding no problems, so they kept telling me that there was nothing to worry about. His heart kept beating irregularly, though, so I pressed that something was wrong. Finally, I was taken to the children's hospital's cardiologist, connected to the hospital that I was in. They did an ultrasound to check our donor's heart. The doctor told us that everything seemed to be fine, and there was nothing to be concerned about at this point.

TUMMERS: After a few days of bed rest, lots of medications (even in the middle of the night), and some serious stress, we met again with Dr. R. He scanned me, and it quickly became obvious that things weren't what he hoped they'd be. It had indeed been a full rupture, as Cameron's fluid was now less than half of what it was at admission. The real fear began with two phrases: "We really needed to get this baby one more week," and "Now we need to discuss a birth plan". We met with the neonatologists twice, to discuss what birth at 27 weeks meant, particularly for Cameron, who was so very tiny for his gestational age (his estimated weight was 650 grams, which put him below the 3rd percentile). We also met with the social worker again, to discuss our concerns, prepare for the arrival of our boys and express our wishes for that moment.

CHRISTMAN-SCHARER: On Friday, I had a perinatal appointment; I was 27 weeks. Baby A still had 3.5 cm of fluid and Baby B 4.5 cm, after they took out 1.7 liters of fluid. I had single contraction. My cervix was still ok. I had bronchitis that week, so I was on an antibiotic.

On Monday (27 weeks, 4 days), I went to perinatal again. Baby A's fluid was 3.5 cm and Baby B's was 5.7 cm. We saw Baby A's bladder again. On Tuesday, I had a 3- hour glucose test. Yuck! On Wednesday (27 weeks, 6 days), at the appointment with the perinatal group, they did a fluid check. Baby A had 4 cm and Baby B had 5 cm. We did not see Baby A's bladder this time. On Thursday, I had a regular ob-gyn appointment. I had gained a total of 31.8 lbs. by then. There was sugar in my urine, but the heartbeats were good, and my glucose came back ok.

REBILAS: Another week of ultrasounds and stress tests.

DILLE: At the ultrasound appointment that week, Cara measured in the 54th percentile, which was great since she was our donor twin. She looked great on her scan; still no signs of hydrops or anemia, and a strong heartbeat. She weighed about 2 ½ pounds.

BRAY: Another week down -- one more to go!

FLETCHER: Monday, May 19th, 2008 was a day we will never forget. I hadn't slept all night, since the pain from the contractions was so intense. I tried taking hot baths to make them go away; I leaned over the tub at one point, crying and praying, waiting for Scott to get home. Scott's dad watched Austin so Scott

could take me to the hospital. I knew in my heart this
would be the girls' birthday.

We went to the hospital, got checked in, and
waited for Dr. L. to come and do an ultrasound. I remember calling my Aunt RoRo, and asking her to call
my sister-in-law, Tiffany. I couldn't remember my
mom's work number, but Tiffany called my brother,
Mikey, who reached Mom at work. Scott called his
family, as well. I had contractions throughout the ul-
tra sound, and when the doctor took the probe out,
my water broke!!

We were so nervous because he said we
couldn't do a vaginal delivery. Dr. B. didn't want to
take any chances, so within minutes I was on my way
to the OR. Mikey and Mom got there just in time to
find out I was having an emergency C-Section. Mikey
took off to get Dad and Tiffany. I think they were as
pale as I was. There was a nurse, Pam, who held my
hand the whole time and cried along with me. I had
never had a C-Section before, nor had I seen so many
people in one room. I remember thinking, "When am
I going to wake up?!" Scott was by my side as Dr. B.
got started. When I heard Dr. B. say, "Oh Man!", and
then ,"Shit" when he opened me up, I thought, "Oh
no! What is wrong?" I could feel pressure from them
pulling one of the babies out and when they did, Dr.
B. said, "Is that the baby with the heartbeat?" I shut
down right there. Scott wiped my tears for me.

They placed Abby in her little bed. All I could
see was her hand and foot, sticking up from her lifeless little body, no movement, no crying. I thought,
"When is this nightmare going to end?" Then they
brought Ally over for us to see before they took her to

NICU. She had one little eye open, her tiny little face looking back at mine. Then they asked me if I wanted to see Abby. I couldn't do it. I just couldn't do it. I knew that Abby was ok in Heaven, in God's arms. I knew she felt how much I love her.

I had never been through this before and didn't know how to cope, so I just shut down, and turned my emotions off. I was so physically and emotionally tired, but felt I had to be strong for everyone around me. If I broke down then, I didn't know how we would keep it together. I guess that is how I justified to myself that it was ok, but not seeing Abby is something I will regret until the day I die. I did see their placenta and cords. I had never seen a cord that thin and tiny.

They got me fixed up and took me back to my room. Our family and friends were there, and I thought, "Where did all of you guys come from?" It had all happened so fast. It was like a dream from which I would soon wake.

Dr. B. came in to talk to me. He said that half of my uterus had flipped over from all the fluid I had lost during the pregnancy, so when he opened me up, he thought I had only half of a uterus. The placenta was really bad; no blood had passed through the cord to Ally since Abby had passed, and Ally's cord had a knot, right at her belly button. Dr. L., Ally's NICU Doctor, came in then to discuss what to expect from Ally, the NICU and the critical first 72 hours.

Later, I was in my hospital room alone and there was a knock on the door. A nurse walked in with a baby. She said, "Here is your baby." I remember looking at her, saying, "My baby is in NICU." She said, "I am so sorry -- wrong room." I broke down.

Before going home, Scott and I left my room, walked to the elevator, and went down to NICU to see Ally. We were so down that day, but Heather, Ally's nurse, said, "It looks like you guys need a pick me up." We got to hold Ally for the first time. She was 3 days old, and it felt like I was holding nothing, but there was this little life in my arms. Three months too early, but life. God knew we needed to hold her that day.

I left the hospital on May 22nd, 2008, with no babies. One daughter was fighting for her life, and I had to plan the other's funeral. Words cannot express the emotions we felt at that time.

Allyson Jean Fletcher was born at 3:15pm, May 19th, 2008, weighing 1 lb. 11.5 oz. She was 13 inches long.

Abbigail Laken Fletcher was born at 3:16pm, May 19th, 2008, weighing-2 lbs. 1.6oz.She was 11.5 inches long.

BRUCE: On August 28, 2007, we went for yet another ultrasound with the Maternal Fetal Medicine doctor. We were at 27 weeks 2 days gestation. Jordyn weighed 1.5 lbs. and Taylor weighed 2.13 lbs. The MFM decided that it was time to receive a series of steroid shots, to help build the twins' lungs in preparation for early delivery.

However, rather than deliver the twins, my OB stated that he wanted me to reach 32 weeks gestation, and that he was going to Italy for his "much needed"

vacation! So, during my 28th and 29th weeks of pregnancy, I went without being seen by my OB or MFM.
I did have a consultation with a pediatric neurologist
regarding Jordyn's hydrocephalus. The neurologist
confirmed the diagnosis of hydrocephalus, but said
that it was mild, and that as soon as Jordyn was stable
after delivery, a shunt would be placed to drain the
fluid from her head. The consultation with the neurologist gave us hope for the first time.

22

Week 28

HADDIGAN: Two hours into week 28, the one everyone wanted us to reach, I woke up with contractions. The doctors checked my water and it had broken; it was time! By the time my husband got there, they were ready to wheel me into the prep room for the c-section.

There were no cries immediately after the twins entered the world. The nurses brought them each to the area that had been prepared. They worked on them for what seemed like forever before announcing that they were wheeling our boys away, to the NICU, and they would call us with an update shortly. I didn't even get to see them before they were taken away.

TUMMERS: Another ultrasound showed good growth in Cameron; he was up to over 750 grams. We had a very scary NICU tour, a reality check for us.

Dr. R. met with us twice to discuss Cameron's growth and fluid levels. He assured us that all was going well and that although he was small, he had been developing as he should, so his lungs would be perfect for a 28-weeker. He also told us that they would be watching for any indication that Cameron was in stress, but that so far everything looked great. They put me on the list to be transferred, as soon as a bed was available at a hospital closer to home.

The social worker brought us some beautiful blankets and outfits for our boys, knit by volunteers.

It was important to me to have matching blankets for my twin sons. I was having such a tough time dealing with the loss right then, away from home, with no family or friends around. I cried a lot, and spent lots of time writing and blogging.

At the end of the week, I was transferred to London (about an hour from home) and had good growth ultrasounds -- almost 1000 grams now! I met with my doctor, Dr. G. He was very concerned about the risks to Cameron posed by the septostomy (the hole in the membrane separating Cameron and Cole), as it allowed the cords to entangle and compress. So, I had a very lengthy ultrasound, with two techs and a doctor, to check this along with the usual growth and flow rates. One of the sweetest comments I'd heard yet came during this ultrasound; the tech described Cameron's position as "gently hugging his brother, Cole". I almost cried.

I got to see my older boys again. It was very sweet and comforting, as were the more frequent visits from friends.

CHRISTMAN-SCHARER: On Friday, I had an appointment with Perinatal for my non-stress test and a fluid check. I was officially 28 weeks on the dot. Baby A had 3.7 cm and Baby B had 9.4 cm; the fluid had gone back up. They estimated Baby A's weight at 1 lb., 5 oz. and Baby B's at 2 lbs. 11 oz. They then gave us two choices: we either let Baby A die in utero, or deliver both babies then, giving them both a fighting chance. I could never let my baby die in utero if I could give her a chance, so we decided to deliver. Weirdly, I was exactly 28 weeks, which was our goal. It was surreal.

The doctors told me to go home and get ready; they would call to schedule my c-section. I couldn't go home and rest, so my boyfriend and I went to the bank and to get some groceries. I called the father of my two older boys, and asked him to get them at daycare, since I'd be in the hospital and it was his weekend anyway. My mother-in-law was already at our house, watching our 1 year old, Reid. While we were grocery shopping, the doctor's office called. They told me not to eat anything and to be at the hospital at 3pm. Good thing they called, because we were going to get something to eat! Instead, we went home and packed Reid to stay at Granny's, grabbed my things, and went to daycare to see Tyler and Alex. We told them that their dad would pick them up, and that we were going to have the babies.

After we arrived at the hospital we waited for the doctor until 5 pm. I had been prepped, but I was starving and kept asking for food. It never entered my mind that anything bad was going to happen. We were very optimistic that everything would be good with the girls. It had to be since I had done everything I could to save them.

At 5:39 pm, Baby A, Karlyn Nicole, was born weighing 1 lb., 4 oz. She was just 12 inches long. Her apgar score was 7 at 1 minute, and 7 at 5 minutes. She was even breathing on her own, but didn't make a sound. She was so tiny, and pure white due to all of her blood going to her sister. At 5:40 pm, Baby B, Kylie Marie, was born weighing 2 lbs., 6 oz. and was just 15 inches long. Her apgar was 7 at 1 minute, and 8 at 5 minutes. She was bright red when born, and very bloated. I got to see each of them quickly, about 30 seconds with each. Thank goodness Karl got a picture of each of them. We never did get a picture of them together, which bothers me to this day. (The only picture I have of them together is one of the ultrasound pictures.) Karlyn was considered a micro-preemie, and she was about 1 ½ months gestational age behind her sister. She was also very anemic; she had at least five blood transfusions after she was born. Karl got to see the girls side by side. When he looked at Karlyn, her sad face seemed to say, "Help me!" They took them to the NICU immediately, and put them on oxygen. My parents were waiting in the hallway, and got to see them side by side, on their way to the NICU.

I went to recovery. When I woke up, they showed me the placenta. It was really messed up. Kylie's side looked normal, but Karlyn's side looked all ground up. We sent it to CHOP for analysis, to aid in the research to put a stop to this horrible disease. They said it was one of the worst cases of twin to twin they had ever seen. Baby A, Karlyn, had a very small share of the placenta; Baby B, Kylie, had the majority of it.

REBILAS: The boys are growing and looking better! In fact, one of our favorite technicians told us that if she didn't know better, she wouldn't think this was TTTS at all given all of the improvements! We were thrilled. What more could you ask for?

HOPE: I experienced one of my postural drop episodes and found myself back at the hospital. In maternity, the usual sort of stuff happened -- lots of questions and monitoring of babies. During the monitoring, a nurse raced out of the room and then hurried back in. After asking me a few questions, she determined I was in the early stages of labor. Dr. C. had been called and was en route to the hospital, but in the meantime, labor had to be stopped. I was admitted and labor was halted. That hospital does not deliver babies before 34 weeks; they are not equipped for or experienced in the delivery. They also discussed the possibility that as soon as the girls were delivered, one or both might have to be flown to the nearest major hospital. I was given another ultrasound, which now showed 4 weeks and 5 days growth difference. I was ordered to spend a couple of days in the hospital, on moderate bed rest. So far, neither baby showed any signs of distress, but both appeared to be very small.

WRIGHT: The doctors continued to monitor my daughter's hydrocephalus. Her brain ventricles had increased a little bit since we first found out, but not too drastically. We met with a neurologist to discuss how our daughter would develop. He was very encouraging.

BRAY: I reached the 28 week mark. The doctors explained that my local hospital, the Royal Glamorgan Hospital (RGH), had contacted him. The special care baby unit there was able to take babies 28 weeks and over. I was discharged that day and placed in the care of the consultants and doctors of RGH's Outpatient Department.

WALLINGTON: At 28 weeks along, they realized that my donor, Lilly, was having decelerations in her heartbeat. That was the beginning of my hospitalization, which lasted until my girls were born. They kept a very close eye on the girls with monitors around the clock, until the day came.

23
Week 29

<u>TUMMERS:</u> I developed some sort of undiagnosed pain. They had no idea why I was having it. It was horrible, kept me up at night, and didn't respond to anything they gave me, which wasn't much -- not even Tylenol, for fear it would mask any signs of infection, like fever. After a few sleepless nights on IV fluids and monitors, they decided to try Tylenol and Ativan to help me sleep. Thankfully, about a week after it began, the pain was gone.

We met with neonatology again. We were filled with such hope to learn that Cameron was now at no more risk of infant mortality than a full-term baby. Obviously, there were still numerous areas of concern due to all that had happened, but the doctors in both the NICU and Antenatal were both very optimistic.

I met my new social worker and broke down on a HUGE scale. It was the first I'd discussed my guilt, and what I really felt in my heart. It was a very tough few days… again!

<u>LIGHT:</u> When I was 29 weeks pregnant, we went for a routine ultrasound with Dr. R. and encountered yet another dilemma, Toxemia. My blood pressure was so high I was admitted without delay, and doctors debated what to do with the babies and me. Most of the OBs wanted to deliver the babies right away, but doing that meant almost certain death for Oliver. The longer he stayed in the womb, the better his chances, and we weren't ready to give up on him.

For three weeks, we waited. While medication kept my blood pressure stable, doctors came and went with different ideas about what was going to happen. I received a non-stress test on the babies twice a day, and daily ultrasounds. Almost every day someone would try to convince me to deliver Sebastian, at the risk of Oliver's life, but Dr. R. would say that everything was fine and we should just wait.

MORGAN: Oops, my water broke! My husband sped us to the ER, where I was told I would probably deliver. A doctor informed me about the developmental issues preemies may incur when born that early.

REBILAS: Hard to believe we made it to 29 weeks! The doctors were all amazed and started talking about getting us to 34 weeks instead of 32! We were in awe! When I left my appointment, I was so happy I just rejoiced. When I got home, I made the usual calls to the grandparents, letting them know how the boys were, and that I was laying down for a nap. I was woken up by the phone ringing; it was the clinic. The new doctor, Dr. M., had checked my scans and decided that I should have the boys the next day! I asked if they were kidding. They told me to get my things together and get to the hospital as soon as possible, so that they could prep me for my C-section. It was so surreal. I called my husband, and told him he had to come home. I got the sitters lined up, and called my closest friends to tell them the big news! As it turned out, the doctor felt that our recipient's stomach was too distended. He had watched a mom lose both children after displaying this symptom.

HOPE: The next few weeks were full of lots of rest, trying to relax, constant doctor's appointments, and ultrasounds. In every ultrasound, Jorja seemed to be dropping off in growth. Doctors advised that at this stage, it was too late to do anything, and in hindsight they should have looked at surgery earlier on. It was very distressing to think that doctors, treating me, had so very little information about TTTS.

BRAY: I was closely monitored by the RGH. I attended twice weekly uss, and daily ctg`s. The twins were growing almost symmetrically, and although my donor twin was without any fluid, his development was lovely.

BRUCE: September 13, 2007 came and I was 29 weeks 4 days. We were at Children's Healthcare of Atlanta at Egleston, for an ultrasound with the fetal cardiologist. This was the first ultrasound where Jordyn's doppler was abnormal, but her heartbeat was around 145 beats per minute. During the ultrasound, I began to feel lightheaded and my mother, who was present along with my husband, mentioned that I looked flushed. She insisted that my blood pressure be checked. The cardiologist acquiesced, and my blood pressure was 175 over something that I can't remember now. My mother insisted that I go to the delivering hospital. The cardiologist was reluctant, but after a phone call to my MFM (not my OB, because he was on vacation in Italy), she told my mother and husband to take me in.

I checked into Atlanta Medical Center's Labor and Delivery and was placed in a triage room, where the nurses hooked up the fetal monitors. They found Taylor's heartbeat right away, but couldn't find

Jordyn's. They brought in the ultrasound equipment to find her, and that's when we saw her heart. Jordyn's heartbeat was so weak that it looked like the flutter of a small butterfly. In seconds, my triage room was filled with nurses, residents and doctors from the NICU. I was prepped and rushed into the operating room for an emergency c-section, so that the NICU could try to save Jordyn. I don't remember falling asleep, but I do remember waking up in recovery, to a room full of sad faces. I remember my nurse asking my family, "Does she know yet?", but I did. No one had to say it. Jordyn was in Heaven.

I had the courage to look at the labor and delivery comments; here is what I found:

"Called for Stat C section of twins with fetal HR abnormalities. Twin A with known hydrocephalus, twins examined earlier in the day by pediatric cards and found to both have HR of 145. Mother presented to hospital after 'feeling ill' and reporting increase in blood pressure to primary OB, who referred for further evaluation at L and D Dept. Upon admission, low variable to no cardiac activity found in Twin A. Twin A delivered w/o HR or resp. drive. Twin A unable to be resuscitated and died in delivery room. Twin B delivered from separate amniotic bag immediately following Twin A. Initial small cry by infant with poor color and tone noted. Placed on radiant warmer and had immediate decrease in HR with resp. effort. HR decreased to less than 60 by 1 min despite stim and then PPV. PPV was continued with adequate ventilation and chest compressions started. HR rose to above 100 by 5 minutes of age after less than 1 min of chest compressions and over 4 total minutes of PPV. Respiratory effort remained intermittent. Tone and color no improvement although reflex present. Infant intubated by RT with ETT placement checked by auscultation by 10 minutes of age. PPV continued via ETT. Tone continued to decrease and color and reflex continued to improve. By 15 minutes of age, infant was stable for transport via isolette to SNUR for further care."

24
Week 30

TUMMERS: Enjoyed some home cooking from an aunt who lives near the hospital, and finally got to escape for a few hours, on an outing with my boys and husband. Tons of jokes were told that week, as I met with the hospital dietician who said I needed to gain a lot of weight. I was so overweight, yet hadn't gained enough in the pregnancy… what a laugh that was to me!

MORGAN: Yes! Still in the hospital on bed rest, we found fluid was growing around Jadon.

DILLE: All of our appointments for Cara have gone well to this point. The doctor says he is fairly confident that we will make it to full term before we deliver. This was great news for us!

DOBBS: On November 15, 2005, we started the once a week appointments. I had some swelling in my feet and hands but not enough to worry about. One of the babies was 3 pounds 7 oz. and the other was 3 pounds 4 oz. The doctor said the fluid level was a little low and I was to go for a stress test tomorrow first thing. We did the first stress test November 16th, and one of the babies was not moving very well.

25
Week 31

TUMMERS: Some changes in my fluid loss this week; it is tinged with blood. Not too worrisome, except that Cameron's heart rate was elevated as well. As there were some contractions as well, they did a few hours of monitoring, but things settled and he remained inside and healthy. The belief was that my uterus was becoming irritated, and I was again told that the doctors did not expect my pregnancy to proceed for much longer.

A few days later, I had measurable contractions and again ended up on the monitor for hours, but again nothing progressed. Cameron's growth ultrasound showed a HUGE gain in only three weeks: 2lbs. 2oz. He now weighed 3lbs. 10oz.

MORGAN: My 2nd week in the hospital, my membranes sealed and Jadon was looking great. I was able to go home, but had to stay on bed rest and could not go back to work.

BRAY: On Saturday, May 30th, I was getting ready to visit my in-laws when the pain started. I was having contractions. We grabbed my notes and headed for the labor ward. I was so scared. I knew my babies were coming. They were still very young - 9 weeks early! I was frightened for my donor baby, since he had been without fluid for such a long time. Were his lungs mature enough? Would he get through this? They prepared me to have a c-section that afternoon. At 5:18pm, my donor twin, Oliver, was born. I didn't hear a cry and they didn't show him to me. I silently started to panic. I looked at Gareth and could see the worry in his eyes. He just looked at me, smiled, and said, "It's ok." At 5:21pm, my recipient, Thomas, was born. When I heard the cry, the tears rolled down my face. They brought him to me and let me kiss his sweet little face before he was taken to SCBU. Then, I was approached by a midwife. "Twin 1 is very, very sick," she explained. "They are doing everything they can for him, but he is critical." My heart sank and I couldn't talk. I just cried.

They took me back to the ward, where I had to wait for 8 hours before they let me see my boys. I was prepared, before I entered the ward, to see that Oliver (twin 1) was still "being worked on"; I wouldn't be allowed to see him, since the doctors were very busy with him. As I entered the high dependency room, I could see four doctors standing around an incubator. It was my Oliver. I caught a glimpse of his tiny little body, and he was grey! There were tubes everywhere; he had bilateral chest drains, and a ventilator breathing for him. The doctor approached me and introduced himself as Dr. Al-M, a neo- natal consultant. Though it was his day off, he had been told about Oliver and came in to help save my baby. I could not thank this man enough. He explained that Oliver was very sick; his lungs were not matured, so he was not able to breathe on his own. He said, "Oliver's been a little fighter, raging against the ventilator, trying his hardest to breathe by himself." Trying to breathe by himself, Oliver had caused both of his lungs to collapse, hence the chest drains. They had had to paralyze Oliver, to stop him from fighting; he needed to rest and let the machines do the work for him. I was allowed to sit with him, his tiny little body so still and motionless, covered in lines and tubes. I felt helpless.

I had done everything I could to save my babies, so now it was up to God.

<u>OROSZ:</u> I had a doctor's appointment at 31 weeks and everything looked good. The Dopplers were normal, so I was told not to worry. I was having what I thought were Braxton Hicks contractions; my belly would get so tight that one of the babies' little bottoms would stick out.

Then, at 31 weeks 5 days, my water broke at 2 am. I woke my husband, shocked. All I kept saying was, "This isn't right -- they aren't supposed to be born yet! It's too early!" We rushed to the hospital, an hour away. They admitted me, halted labor with magnesium, and gave me two steroid shots within 48 hours. The magnesium really made me sick and "out of it". I felt helpless, and was reminded of TTTS, even though I thought we would make it to the end (or at least 37 or 38 weeks.) I knew the average gestation age of babies who had the laser surgery, but since everything was looking great, I had put the TTTS in the back of my mind.

<u>DOBBS:</u> November 23, 2005, I had another ultrasound. I had some swelling in my feet and hands, so I went for more blood work, and was told to go home and put my feet up.

26
Week 32

TUMMERS: Some scary and stressful times that
week, as Cameron's MCA (which measures the rate of
blood flow in the brain, basically indicating blood
volume and anemia) was high, bordering on prob-
lematic. No one seemed concerned but Geoff and I,
and no one could explain why it had happened. The
consensus was that he couldn't be anemic, nor did
other possible explanations fit. That meant more
tests, scans, and finally a face to face meeting with
some of my team (which, in the four weeks I'd been
there, had so far never happened). A new birth plan
was written, but the stress of each new doctor on
rounds rewriting what had been decided was too
much for me.

LIGHT: One normal Saturday, everything changed
drastically. Rob had spent the previous few nights
sleeping in a chair next to my bed, and was desperate
for a good night's sleep in his own bed, so he went
home to relax. It was the night before Mother's Day,
and my nurse and I joked about how funny it would
be if I became a mommy on Mother's Day. Little did I
know!

About a half hour later, I had a blinding head-
ache, and saw "snow" falling in my room. That
night's non-stress test showed that both babies were
in distress, and my blood pressure was climbing by
the minute, despite medication. Both of the on-call
OB's told me that we couldn't extend the pregnancy
any longer, and before I knew it, there we were in the
delivery room. At 1:34 AM, Sebastian Cedric was

born, weighing 3lbs 15oz. Oliver Calvin followed at 1:37am, weighing 1lb 9oz.

WRIGHT: My daughter's hydrocephalus seemed to have stabilized. Due to Sarah's death, the doctors said, most would go into pre-term labor. From the research I had done, I knew that most do go into labor between 30-32 weeks, so I was starting to get worried that Julie Anne would not only have neurological problems, but also breathing problems. I remained on bed rest to prevent pre-term labor.

OROSZ: I was hospitalized for two weeks with ruptured membranes, and scheduled for a c-section at 34 weeks. It was a very long two weeks, back on bed rest. The first few nights in the hospital, I cried. I missed my husband, who couldn't stay with me because he had to be home with our 3 year old who I also missed. They came to visit me as often as they could, but my husband still had to go to work. We couldn't afford him to be off without pay, and he had used all of his vacation days when we were in Philadelphia.

27
Week 33

<u>TUMMERS:</u> MCA remained high, at the top of the threshold for normal. The new MFM on rounds felt this was a concern, as it had been normal the entire time I'd been there. He decided that it was time to book a c-section, and a delivery date was set for the next week.

<u>HOPE:</u> Monday's ultrasound showed some small growth from the previous ultrasound, while Thursday's showed no difference. We knew we were in the danger zone when Jorja stopped growing. Thursday afternoon, after receiving the results, we phoned Dr. C. at home, to inquire about his plan. He calmly replied, "You have an appointment in the morning, so we will talk about it then."

We arrived at 9am, and were led into the doctor's room and informed he was running 5 minutes late. When he did enter, he breezed past, saying, "Hi. I have been to maternity, and I have been to surgery. I have booked you beds and I will see you at 3pm today to get these little girls out." Immediate shock set in. Wow! We were finally going to meet our little girls, that day. Then a dark shadow came over us, as we thought, "Are they going to be alive?"

We arrived at the hospital at 12:30pm and settled into my room while the staff prepared us for what was about to happen. We were fully aware that if either baby came out in less than good condition, an air ambulance was on standby, waiting to take them away. Surprisingly, from the time I got there until I was wheeled into surgery at 3pm, time seemed to fly. I was completely relaxed about having a cesarean, since I had elected to have one very early on. My concern was for my babies.

At precisely 3:30pm on the 4th of July 2003, Chloe Ann Hope was born weighing 4lb. 8oz., and at 3:32pm, Jorja Lee Hope was born weighing 2lb. 4oz.

Chloe was in great condition and breathing on her own. Jorja was born black, but quickly gained color. She was grunting slightly; we were later told this was to prevent her lungs from collapsing. Both girls were quickly taken to the NICU while I was left to recover. I wouldn't see either of them until 9 the next morning.

OROSZ: They gave me two more steroid shots on two days of week 33, as I had developed a very itchy rash all over my body. It was two days before the scheduled c-section.

I had contractions for hours the night before the twins were born. I told the nurses, who said that if the pain got worse or the contractions were 5 minutes apart, they would hook me up to the machine. Finally, it got to the point where I couldn't take the pain and was so tired. I had the nurses hook me up to the machine, but my contractions weren't picking up. It was almost like they didn't believe me, but when they moved the belt further down my belly, sure enough, contractions showed up on the screen. The doctor was called; it was time to deliver. I had to get in touch with my husband, so he could drive to the hospital and be there for the twins' birth. My OB was kind enough to wait for my husband to get there. As soon as he was in the room, he dressed in the paper scrubs, and I was wheeled away to the operating room.

My twins decided to come two days before 34 weeks, on May 15th, at 6:29 am. They weighed 4 lb., 2 oz. I remember lying on the operating table, scared, as we didn't know what the outcome would be. Would their lungs be ok to breathe? Would they be the right weight? I felt a lot of pressure in my chest when they were pulling the babies out. They came out crying, and were rushed to the RICN while they stitched me up. I was happy they were here, and happier to hear them cry! Baby B was delivered first, because he was head down, and Baby A was second because he was in breech. My husband got to hold both of them and I got to see them and kiss them. They were perfect! My mother brought our 3 year old to meet his little brothers the day they were born. He was such a proud big brother.

DOBBS: December 05, 2005, I had to go to the emergency room because I could not feel my legs and was having trouble remembering things. They called in a neurologist, Dr. K., who did a full neurological exam and said he couldn't find any reason for these symptoms. I spent the next couple of hours resting while they monitored the babies.

On December 8, 2005, another stress test and then off to see Dr. P. During the stress test, one of the babies was not moving as well as the other. I started to worry at this point, since I did not feel well and was having trouble sleeping. Dr. P. told me one them was 4 pounds 8 ounces, and the other was 5 pounds even. He instructed that if I went into labor, I should go straight to the Emergency room, where he would meet us.

WALLINGTON: September 12th 2005 was the day that the doctors told me I would be delivering my daughters. Lilly had been struggling in the night and had had many decelerations in her heartbeat.

The day I had fought so long and hard for the last 7 ½ months had finally come. They would be born at 33 weeks. I shook with fear and anticipation. I thanked God endlessly for getting us to this point and prayed for Him to carry us through what was to come. As I lay in bed, thinking of my children's birthday, something dawned on me. It was Sept 12th, the exact same day I had miscarried the year before, with the same doctors there to help me through. They were all astonished at this, and truly felt blessed to be a part of it. I felt as though God was giving me back the twins I had lost. It was very ironic, yet very clear to me at the same time. Sometimes God takes things from us so we can truly and deeply appreciate other moments and people in our lives. It may not happen when we want it to; it can come slowly or swiftly. But this I know, God never wants us to suffer. He wants us to be strong in our Faith in Him, and to let him lead us where He may, even though we may feel we are in the dark, alone.

Our daughters, Lilly and Londyn, were born at 6:13 and 6:14 p.m. on September 12th, 2005. They were beautiful. Lilly was 2 lbs. 3oz and 13 inches long. Londyn was 4 lbs. and 16 inches long.

28
Weeks 34 and 35

TUMMERS: Tons of emotions and stress this week, leading up to delivery day. My social worker was on holiday, so that didn't help. We made a plan before she left, but I was very sure it wouldn't be followed. Geoff met with the funeral home and delivered the small casket his father had made to have Cole transported to the crematorium in. All in all, it was a week filled with sadness and tears.

We met again with the neonatologist, and got the worst case and most likely scenarios painted for us. It was assumed that Cameron would need some breathing support, most likely CPAP. It was projected that he would be well over 5 lbs., and would probably need an NG tube for one week, then orally feed.

Then, on February 26th, we welcomed our sons, Cameron Cole Gregory and Cole Edward Ryan, into the world.

WRIGHT: Julie Anne's hydrocephalus was still stable. We discussed scheduling the c-section, and made arrangements for Sarah's burial. Sarah's body was starting to deflate. It was very hard to see her wither on the ultrasound.

DILLE: I believe we were at week 34 when one of my weekly ultrasounds turned into a non- stress test. The tech was trying to scan Cara, but she wasn't moving much. Cara didn't wake up after being pushed and poked, so the tech got out a buzzer to try and wake her. That didn't work, either. She would jump when she heard it, but then go back to sleep. The tech was concerned; this meant Cara didn't pass her biophysical profile, so I was sent for the non-stress test. I was monitored for about a half an hour or so, and Cara was moving all over the place. They said things looked great, but they wanted me to come back the next day to do another ultrasound and non-stress test. Cara passed those tests with flying colors, so we were sent home again. I was once again relieved that we had made it another week.

DILLE: At the end of week 35, I was released from the high risk clinic and sent back to my regular OB. I was glad to be back with Dr. B., because I really wanted her to deliver my twins. She had delivered both my older children. I knew her well, and trusted her.

29
Week 36+

MORGAN: At 40.5 weeks, I had to be induced. The amniotic fluid was decreasing and Jadon was on his way. In my mind, I knew I was going to have a healthy baby, but because of all the issues Jadon had faced in utero, I wasn't sure what to expect when I delivered him.

WRIGHT: Julie Anne and Sarah's delivery went very smoothly. We were able to deliver at full term, so there was no need for Julie Anne to go to the NICU. She was doing so well.

DILLE: When I went to my 36 weeks appointment, Dr. B. and I talked about scheduling an induction, and decided on March 31, 2009: 38 ½ weeks. We also discussed what would happen at the delivery. Dr. B. told me that she would schedule special nurses, more capable of handling our difficult delivery, for my induction. She also made an appointment for my husband and me to talk with the chaplain at the hospital where we would be delivering.

I was nervous that week, because my doctor was on vacation. Then I woke up one night and couldn't go back to sleep. I realized that I hadn't felt Cara move in a while, and when I pushed on her to try and rouse her, she wouldn't move. I drank some water and waited an hour. I changed positions and tried other tricks to wake her, but still she didn't move. So, my husband and I went to the hospital to check on her. I was hooked up to the monitors, and shortly thereafter, Cara started moving around. She was not as active as usual, so I stayed at the hospital a few more hours so she could be monitored. Everything looked fine at that point, so we were released and sent home. We were back twice more that week with contractions. I just hoped that I wouldn't go into labor until my doctor got back. She returned two days after my last trip to labor and delivery.

At 38 weeks 5 days, my husband and I headed to the hospital to be induced. I was no stranger to induction, since both of my other pregnancies had ended that way. The nurses all knew our situation, and were very sympathetic. They started the pitocin and we were on our way. Dr. B. came in around 9:30 to break my water, which put me into full labor. I don't remember much about my labor, but it was fairly uneventful. I finally asked for an epidural around 1:30, when I was about 5 centimeters dilated. By the time the anesthesiologist finished with the epidural, I was ready to push. I only pushed for about five minutes before Cara was born. I was worried that she was not going to be okay, but my husband calmed my fears and told me that she was. She was beautiful, though I remember thinking that she was pretty small. Dr. B. put her on my chest while she helped deliver Tessa. I kept asking my husband if she was out yet, and what she looked like. We had spent 4 ½ months wondering what Tessa would look like when she was delivered, so I was anxious to finally see her. I finally got to see and hold her. She looked better than the doctors had prepared us for. She was very small, weighing only about a half a pound. She had been close to 2 pounds at the time of the surgery, when she died. Her body was flattened, but we could make out almost all of her features. It was amazing how much she actually resembled Cara.

They both had long fingers and toes, and their facial features looked remarkably similar, given the condition of Tessa's body. I liked the fact that I could tell they were identical.

My parents were able to see Tessa, as were our greatest family friends, who had lost their 18 year old daughter 3 years before. I wanted them to meet my sweet Angel, Tessa. I took pictures with both my girls. It was very important to me to have that, and I knew it would be important to Cara, too, when she got older. We spent a few hours with Tessa in our room, but then it was time to say our final goodbyes. Our older children (who we didn't allow to see Tessa because we thought it would be too much for them) were anxious to see Cara and me.

DOBBS: I went to Dr. P. once a week and had stress tests done. By that point in my pregnancy, I hurt everywhere and did nothing but try to sleep. On December 25, 2005, the swelling I had experienced spread to my legs and face. I felt sick to my stomach all day, and I was so tired. There was less movement in both of the babies that day. I went to the doctor on December 27, 2005, and had gained 17 pounds since my previous appointment. Dr. P. said he would have to do a C-section, on December 28, 2005, at 12:00 noon. When I arrived in the operating room, there was a pediatrician by the name of Dr. M., a team of nurses for each of the girls, and a team of interns who had asked if they could see twins born. At 12:30, Baby A, Ashlee Kale Dobbs, was delivered at 5 pounds 15 oz., and at 12:31, Baby B, Emilee Mae Dobbs, was delivered at 6 pounds 14 oz.

30
The NICU Stay: The First 24 Hours

<u>BRUCH:</u> My very first visit to the NICU to see my own children is something I will never forget. (I was there years before, seeing a friend's child.) I looked around and saw 30 babies, all on an assortment of machines. I was taken to two isolates. My boys were so small, but alive. Vincent was 11 oz. and Thomas was 1 lb.3 oz. They gripped 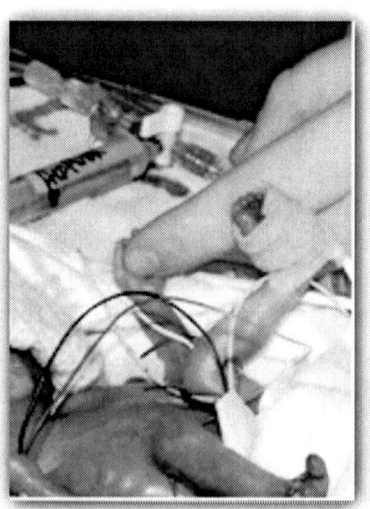 my finger. I even heard Thomas cry. I didn't know a 24-week baby could cry; some 34 week babies can't even do that! I saw each of their chests rise with each breath they took, and their tiny hearts where quickly fluttering. My boys were each on an oscillator that helped them to breathe. They were small, but they were mine. Within six hours of their birth, we had a makeshift baptism. Vincent's god parents were my brother and sister, Jason and Dawn. Thomas's god parents were Matthew and his wife, Amber.

That night around 1:50 am, Vincent passed away. They had given me a sleeping pill, so it seemed like a dream. When I woke up, I felt as though the world was changed forever. The nurse came and asked if I wanted to hold my son. I called my husband and family in to hold Vincent. He deserved to be held; every child deserves to be held and told that they are loved. We cried, but knew Thomas was alive.

HADDIGAN: We didn't hear anything for 12 hours, then, we were finally able to go and see our boys. They were in separate areas, so we couldn't see them together. They had tubes and wires everywhere. They were tiny - Riley, our donor, was 2 lbs. 9 oz., and Logan, our recipient, was 2 lbs. 7 oz.

TUMMERS: We were very fortunate. Cameron required only free flow oxygen at birth; his apgar was 8 at birth and 9 at five minutes. He was doing GREAT!!! The only issues we encountered were low glucose levels, high bilirubin, and a HUGE problem gaining weight since he was very small for his gestational age, only 4 lbs. 1.5 oz. (the 10th percentile, making him IUGR, as well)

LIGHT: Sebastian spent three weeks in the Mount Sinai NICU, with a case of jaundice, and a few days of particularly shallow breathing. He then spent one week in the Level 2 Nursery, before being transferred to Guelph General Hospital for a week. On June 23rd, we brought him home, weighing a little over 5 lbs.! Oliver spent 2 months in the Mount Sinai NICU, where he endured a blood transfusion, a PIC Line, and was on and off the CPAP.

CHRISTMAN-SCHARER: Karl and my parents got to see the girls before I did. I couldn't get out of bed for a long time, due to the spinal I'd had. When I finally saw them, they were in incubators, side by side, and were so tiny. They had tubes and lines all over them. They actually looked like baby birds lying in a nest.

They told us Kylie was doing very well and that pre-mature girls thrive better than boys. That was another positive thing to hold onto. Later that night everyone went home. I told Karl to go as well and get some rest, because he wouldn't get a lot in the hospital. He planned to go to work the next day.

Later that night, they came and told me that Karlyn was very sick and needed a special machine, called an oscillator. Theirs was in use, so they called around to the local hospitals, but they were all being used. They wanted to send her to St Christopher's, which is about two hour's drive from where we were. I said of course and signed the form. Anything that we could do to help her! They took her at about 5 the next morning. I saw her a few times before they took her, but wasn't allowed to hold her. I watched them transport her. It was raining that night; I remember it so well. It was also the last time I saw my angel, Karlyn, alive.

I had called Karl about moving her, and he said he was alright with it. Now, we don't know if we made the right decision. Could they have treated her where we were? Would we have had more time with her? Karl and his parents went the next day, to see her and talk to her doctors. They said she was critical, but stable. They had her sedated because she was in a lot of pain. They were giving her medicine to open up her blood vessels, since they were tiny and stuck together, due to her not getting enough blood.

MORGAN: When my membranes ruptured at 29 weeks, I was told I would be taking a trip to the NICU before my survivor was born. Luckily, we never made it – my membranes sealed back up. I was very nervous and scared that having the baby so early would mean developmental issues for my son. I remember staying strong, because that's all I could do.

REBILAS: I had the boys at 29 weeks 5 days. They weighed 2 pounds 4 ounces, and 3 pounds 8 ounces. Our donor, baby B, was born first and all of a sudden known as baby A. I know that seems like a small thing, but after explaining to friends and family about baby A and baby B, now that they were reversed, well, it was interesting. Our boys had few to no issues in the NICU, all they needed was to grow. During the first week, though, one would do well and the other would have a rough go, and the next day, it would flip-flop. It really helped keep our spirits up that one was always doing well. Our donor spent 9 weeks in the NICU, and our recipient 6 weeks there.

HOPE: Since we were at a smaller hospital, the NICU was just part of the newborn nursery, but with more equipment and the most senior nurses. Everyone seemed excited to have the girls there. Chloe was released out onto the ward, with me taking on her full care, after only a day. Unknown to us, Jorja would spend the next 13 weeks there. I tried to spend as much time with Jorja as I could, but found it very difficult when I was not allowed to touch or care for her. The nursing staff had never cared for a baby Jorja's size, so it was a learning experience for them. Fortunately, the pediatrician caring for her had just moved there from the major children's hospital in Sydney, so he was very up to date.

It was only on the advice of another mother (whose little boy had just been transferred from Sydney, born 5 months earlier at less than 1lb) that we were finally allowed to hold Jorja and participate in her care. While that mother was educating the nurses on how the big hospitals did things, she was also an immense support for David and me. Day 5, she suggested we dress Jorja in some clothes, making her the little person she is, not just a thing in a humidi crib. It was advice like this that helped us cope with what was happening around us.

BRAY: They took me to Thomas. "He's doing really well," they told me, "We have given him c-pap, just so that he can rest, but he has been pulling it off and is maintaining his oxygen levels fine." Thomas was sleeping on his tummy, with his little bottom in the air. He was very pink, but so gorgeous. Oliver was taken off the paralyzing medication; his bloods were improving, and he was a lot more stable. My two beautiful boys - I was so proud.

OROSZ: I was so heartbroken when I went to the RICN (regional intensive care nursery) to see them; they had NG tubes, oxygen, and IVs in their little heads. It was the saddest day; I didn't even get to hold them on their birthday. The nurses were very informative, telling me the babies were doing well and would be off oxygen by the next day. I hated going into the RICN; it was so depressing and sad. I wanted so badly for my boys to come home and be with us! If I wasn't there with them, I would call to check their weight gain and ask how they were doing. The nurses told me what my boys needed to do in order to come home: suck, breathe, maintain body temperature outside of the incubator, and gain weight. Then they needed to be able to sit in their car seats for an hour, maintaining respiration and body temp. They were slow eaters for a while. They held their body temperature, and did everything they needed to, so they were moved out of the incubators. Some of the nurses were more positive than others, but the boys were released after 10 days.

FLETCHER: The doctors and nurses in NICU were amazing! They were there for us from day one. We were so scared, but they would reassure us that Allyson was going to be ok. They explained everything to us: how the NICU worked, what to expect in the coming days, and that this would be the most emotional roller coaster ride we had ever been on. And it was.

I remember the first day and night she was in the NICU. They rolled me down, in my bed, to see her for the first time. All I could see were tiny little feet, the tiniest little feet I had ever seen. It was hard to see her hooked up to all the machines. We wanted to help, but there was nothing we could do but pray! I had seen a miracle that day, a little girl with such fire and fight inside of her.

DOBBS: Ashlee was very pale, and so weak that she could not cry. Emilee was maroon, and not breathing on her own, so she too was not crying! Dr. M. began to work on them as I was wheeled into recovery. An hour later, I was wheeled into the nursery and our lives changed forever. Dr. M. said that Emilee had to be transferred to another hospital, better equipped to handle her case. Her hematocrit was very high; she would have to have a blood transfusion. We had enough time to have her baptized before she was sent to Allegany General Hospital in Pittsburgh. Michael and his mother, Ada, went with her. I stayed in Wheeling with Ashlee, who was severely anemic and jaundiced. The nurses allowed me to hold her for a few seconds before they took her, started her on an iron drip, and put her on a bilirubin blanket for the rest of the night. They gave me a sedative, so I slept.

WALLINGTON: The girls were in the NICU for 8 long weeks. It was another long, hard process for them, but we had won our fight. My girls were in this world and healthy, just small. It was hard to see them in their little beds with tubes and oxygen.

JELLEY: Ellina was breathing with the help of only a CPAP, although she would have to be intubated later. She was the smallest thing I had ever seen in my life. The doctor said she was doing really well.

The nurse brought Ellianna to me and I held her for a little while. She was so perfect, although so small that her head was about the size of an egg. The nurse was afraid to bring Emmalin to me, because she was so squished. I realize the nurse was just trying to protect me, but they were my babies, and though it saddens me that they had any pain, I don't care how it made them look.

BRUCE: The first 24 hours were very blurry. My uterus began to contract while I was still in recovery. I was in so much pain that the doctor prescribed something stronger than morphine, which made me feel even loopier and everything seem more dream-like. The recovery nurse asked if I wanted to see Jordyn, and I told her that I wanted to wait until I was in my private room, alone with my family. I didn't know at the time that my husband had already seen and held Jordyn. Apparently, the nurses brought her to him shortly after she passed away, while I was still under in the operation room. He asked them to take her away until I was ready.

She was so beautiful and perfect. Everyone got to hold and love Jordyn. The nurse took a few Polaroids of her, but looking back, I wish someone had thought to get their digital camera, so we could have more (and nicer) pictures of her. Our family left my husband and me to be alone with Jordyn. We cuddled up on the hospital bed, with her between us. After it grew late, I decided to let Jordyn go and went to the NICU to finally see Taylor.

Taylor had so many wires coming off of her. Nothing could have prepared me to see her in such a state. She was on a ventilator and under jaundice lights. She was so tiny that the bed they had her in looked as if it could just swallow her up. We couldn't hold her because she was on the ventilator, and the nurses didn't want us to touch her a lot. The pain from the c-section grew, and I had to retire for the rest of the night. Taylor remained in NICU for 6 weeks.

31
The Long Days in The NICU

<u>BRUCH:</u> Thomas was doing so well. He did everything that the NICU needed him to do. He had two nurses dedicated to him 24/7. He was on the machines but was taking his own breaths. He had the ventilator, but most of his breaths were his own, and not the machine's. He would move when he heard our voices. He could smile, and make facial expressions. He never looked like he was in pain. He was our fighter, our hope, and he was doing well. I would call or visit him every three hours to check in, but I began to feel like I was forgetting my daughter. How can you parent two children when one is in the hospital and the other is visiting with family members? I felt so bad, but thought it could only get better. It annoyed me to no end when the NICU team called Thomas "sick"; he wasn't sick, HE WAS JUST SMALL!

<u>HADDIGAN:</u> Riley and Logan were perfect, they just had to continue their fight on the outside. On day four, I called first thing, to check how their night had gone. Both were doing all right. Riley would be fed that afternoon, if he continued to show improvement. Logan's oxygen requirements had decreased. They were doing great! We were so happy that morning; everything was going perfectly.

<u>TUMMERS:</u> Cameron lost weight for the first week, so the NG tube remained in place. He was a great nurser, though, and didn't even try to bottle feed until he was 2 weeks old. He was born with significant contractures in all his limbs, and received physio

daily. An interesting thing had happened when he arrived: he had a very large open wound under his arm. It wasn't from the c-section, but rather something in utero. The staff had never seen such a thing, but I was later told that it may very well have been an amnio band. Though it had caused no trouble, there is a scar from the front of his shoulder to the back of it, which he will carry forever.

After 15 days, he was transferred to our local hospital, where he began exclusively feeding orally. He left the hospital at 22 days old, weighing 4 lbs. 12 oz.

LIGHT: Oliver was finally transferred to Grand River Hospital on July 17th, 2 months and 6 days after his birth! He was there for 6 days, then came home with us on July 23rd, weighing 5 lbs. AT LAST!

CHRISTMAN-SCHARER: The day after the girls were born, I was watching them take care of Kylie when she had a reaction to some meds they gave her. The machines were beeping like crazy, but they told us not to worry about that. I was still really drugged up, so when they called other people over to help with her, I didn't realize that anything was seriously wrong. I knew she was sick, but they said this was just a reaction to the meds. Besides, they knew what to do. They kept asking if I wanted to go back to my room and I told them no. Then things started to calm down, and they said she was doing better. Little did I know that while I was sitting there, my daughter's heart stopped. They were able to resuscitate her, thank God, but I had no idea until a year later. They had told Karl, but he told them not to tell me. I think he made a good decision, because she turned out to be ok.

I had the girls Friday evening and got out of the hospital on Monday. We called St. Christopher's a few times a day, to find out what was going on with Karlyn. Nothing was changing, nothing getting worse. They said I needed to get up there, but I had to stay in the hospital for four days. It was also very hard for Karl to get there, having three other kids. It wasn't that we didn't want to see her, it was just hard to get there.

Late Monday afternoon, I went home, rested and saw my three boys. I had never been away from them for that long. We planned to see Karlyn on Tuesday morning, a decision I regret. I should have gone Monday, after I got out of the hospital, but I missed my other kids. If I had known what we were in for on Tuesday, I would not have waited. But my 1 year old missed me and needed me, too, just as the other boys did.

In all, Kylie was in the NICU for 51 days. Both girls were intubated at birth. Though they were breathing on their own some, they needed help. After Karlyn passed away, Kylie improved by leaps and bounds. Karlyn must have given her strength somehow. We were able to touch Kylie the day Karlyn passed away, and soon after, we were able to hold her, bathe her, help change her monitors and feed her through her feeding tube. She was on cpap for about a month, and then on the nasal cannula. She grew every day, getting bigger. Most preemie babies come home after their due dates, but Kylie came home one month before hers, on August 13th. She weighed 4 lbs., 9 oz. She had an apnea monitor until November. They told us, before we left, that she could have physical and mental problems. She saw a heart specialist, hearing specialist and eye specialist. She is now a perfectly healthy 3 year old. She has no signs of problems and is doing the same or better than her friends at daycare. We are so blessed to have her with us.

After Karlyn passed away, I made up a song for Reid and Kylie, about their sister. Sung to the tune of "All day, all night, Angels watching over me my lord", her song goes "All day, all night, sister Karlyn watching over me. All day, all night, sister Karlyn watching me." They both loved listening to me sing it when I rocked them. Sometimes, I catch them singing the song and it makes me smile.

REBILAS: The worst part of the NICU stay was dividing my time. I had a small son at home, who I cared for while my husband was at work. My husband would stop by the hospital on his way home and visit with the boys. Then, when he got home, I went, and often spent hours there. The entire time the boys were in the NICU, I never missed my daily visit. I remember telling one of the nurses that I wouldn't be there at my normal time, but I would be in a little later, and she told me, "Oh, that's fine. You are an 'every day', we know you'll be here." I guess they really keep track of that. One day, I looked at the chart because the nurse hadn't yet given me the update. In it, I read, "Mother called to check on the babies. Father came in to visit at 4:30pm. Both parents appear loving, genuinely concerned and kind." At think that moment, it hit me how blessed we were to be able to see our babies every day. I know there were others who couldn't make that happen. I felt for parents who just had to trust that their babies were being cared for.

HOPE: These 13 weeks in the NICU were some of the hardest I faced. Jorja had settled, and all her little problems, like jaundice, had corrected themselves. David had returned to work, which he found upsetting, but every spare moment he had, he spent in the NICU. I was at home with Chloe, trying to settle her into a routine, and to adjust to mother hood. I spent all my time feeding and settling Chloe, only to pack her up to go spend as much time as possible with Jorja. We were lucky; the NICU staff enjoyed both girls, and it was safe enough to take Jorja out and let her cuddle with Chloe. It was during these cuddles that both girls seemed most content. We had family sporadically, but mostly it was just the two of us. Sometimes, if we weren't too buggered, David would let me sneak off in the night to spend time with Jorja. The first thing we did every morning when we got up was ring to see how her night had been.

BRAY: My grandmother, auntie, and in-laws came to visit. I was happy again; I began to relax a little. My boys are going to be ok, I thought to myself. But then, the following morning, the tables turned again. I asked the midwives to go phone the scbu first thing. She came back and said, "Twin 2 is lovely, but twin 1 is very sick. The doctor would like to talk with you and your partner this morning." When I finally got to speak to the doctor, I was an emotional wreck and could not stop crying. He explained to us that they thought Oliver had perforated his intestine, so he was transferred by ambulance to the University Hospital of Wales, in Cardiff, to be seen by the surgeons. He said we should prepare ourselves for Oliver having surgery. I signed myself out of the post natal ward and followed him to that hospital.

When we arrived at the NICU, we were approached by a locum consultant. He took us into a small room off the unit, where he sat us down and explained their concerns. They thought Oliver had a bleed to his brain, which was confirmed after a USS of his head. He had suffered a grade 3 bleed to the left side of his brain, and a grade 4 to the right side. They were worried he wouldn't make it through the next 24 hours. We sat at his incubator, watching the nurses give him blood transfusion after blood transfusion. He was getting worse, becoming more and more swollen.

The following morning (Tuesday, June 2nd), the doctors suggested we call our family in, since there was nothing more they could do for our son. They were going to have to turn off his ventilator. I was numb. My heart broke more with each word that came out of the doctor's mouth. My Oliver had fought so hard, but he just could not go on. My family came to the hospital and both sets of parents said their tearful goodbyes to their grandson. It was time to turn the ventilator off. I held my son, for the first time, as he died in my arms. I will never forget the pain I felt.

We stayed with Oliver for several hours. I kissed his tiny face a thousand times. I didn't want to let him go, but the time came when the nurse had to take him away from me. I couldn't watch as she walked out of the room. My baby boy was gone. How could I ever get through this?

Thomas came on in leaps and bounds. He stayed at the scbu for a total of 35 days. I can't explain how I felt. It all seems like such a blur. Thomas was perfect, with no major problems other than his size. He needed to put on weight and to feed from a bottle. The nurses were fantastic; they always sat, listened, and comforted me when I cried over Oliver. They had never had a case like ours before. A lot of the staff had never cared for twins with TTTS as severe as ours.

OROSZ: While their ten day in the RICN were hard, leaving the hospital without them was even harder. Driving back there every day was difficult as well, because our 3 year old needed a babysitter most of the time. My mother and grandmother were amazingly supportive through it all. They helped with my toddler and gave me emotional support. Overall, they were very good about taking care of our boys. I cried every single day I went to visit the RICN; it was so hard not being able to have them home with us.

FLETCHER: Ally had her good days and her bad days. She would gain weight and then lose it. I had a talk with her about dieting; I told her she could worry about her weight when she got older, but that now wasn't the time, and she needed every ounce.

I love the doctors and nurses at Holston Valley NICU. No matter if I just wanted to talk, or didn't want to say much, they were there for me. I could call them in the middle of the night, which Scott did often, since he worked the graveyard shift.

Ally came off of the ventilator after three days, which was amazing. She only had one setback; she had gotten staph, and so went back on it for a couple of days. I remember her first bath (we were so afraid we would break her), her first bottle, and her first smile. It was tough being unable to be with her 24/7, but the nurses were wonderful. If something changed, they called us, no matter what time.

I met other parents in the NICU. Some of them didn't get to take their babies home, because they had passed away. I felt so guilty because Ally was doing so well. I thought, God wanted me to see this, to show me that I couldn't have handled watching Abby suffer for one minute. I remember Ally's first bow, and the first time she wore clothes. Going to the NICU became an everyday routine for 74 days, until Ally was finally able to come home! That was the most amazing feeling in the world, but scary at the same time. Preemie babies are not like full term babies. Ally came home with oxygen and a monitor, which scared me to death until I got used to it. The night we left, one of the nurses jokingly told us she wanted joint custody. The staff had been so good to us, they became like family. The morning after Ally came home, I accidentally called the NICU. Heather answered the phone, so I started the normal questions. She started laughing, and I said, "What?" She said, "Honey, you will have to weigh Ally and look to see how she is doing, because she is home with you." We both cracked up. That call is still talked about in the NICU, to this day.

DOBBS: By day two, Michael called to say that Emilee had made it through the night but was very sick. They had already done the first blood transfusion before Michael and Ada got there. They were letting her rest before giving her another one. Dr. M. came in before 6:00 the following morning. He had been on the phone with Dr. S from Pittsburgh, and after going over the pathology report, they thought the girls had twin to twin transfusion syndrome.

By day three, Ashlee was getting stronger and able to eat, though she still spent most of her time under the bilirubin lights. She would stay under them, getting stronger, for two more days. Emilee, on the other hand, had a long road ahead of her. She was given a second blood transfusion; we had to wait for her body to react. On day five, Ashlee was strong enough to come home. We had to take her to Dr. M. once a week, for a month, to make sure her iron was good and that she was not jaundiced. At home, she adjusted well, but while she slept, she would moan and whimper.

WALLINGTON: They had won their fight. Now, all they had to do was grow, and anticipate the abundance of love they would get from their parents.

JELLEY: Ellina was doing really well. She even sucked some breast milk off of a cotton swab, so they gave her some through her feeding tube every 12 hours. She received another chest x-ray, and a scan of her brain to check for bleeds, but everyone was very encouraged by how well she was doing. She gripped my hand with her tiny little fingers and tried to cry, but it sounded like a little mouse squeak.

32
Our survivors

HADDIGAN: Only two days later, Logan had heart surgery to open his thickened ventricle, which was overworked due to the TTTS. The cardiologist said Logan was the smallest baby he'd ever treated. Prior to the surgery, he'd had several "bradies" (bradycardia), and I was scared to death. We walked with them to the operating room, past the nursery where Riley had been just two days before. It hit me like a ton of bricks - what would we do if we lost Logan, too?

Thankfully, he made it through. He was a fighter; within a few days, he was being fed through a tube. There were ups and downs. There were middle-of-the-night phone calls authorizing a pic line, but there were also wonderful moments when he would open his eyes and look at us or hold our finger. The smallest sign of life from him was all we needed to thrill us. He would fuss when the nurses messed with him, so they told us he was feisty, which was a good thing in the NICU. He was moved to the step down unit, where he learned to eat from a bottle. The speech therapist told me not to expect much from him at the first feeding, but I knew better; my boy was an eater! She had a two-ounce bottle and said she'd be thrilled if he ate half an ounce. Logan ate the entire bottle!

After nine weeks, we finally got to go home with our baby. Logan was barely 5 pounds and not even due to be born for another three weeks. Since then, Logan has grown and is happy and healthy. We have had developmental testing and he is right on target. We are still concerned about his heart issues, but hopeful that he will stay strong and continue to improve. We plan to make Logan aware of Riley, as our older son talks about him all the time. He'll always know that he is a twin.

The suffering I watched my oldest son endure was worse than anything I could have imagined. The questions that I had to answer, and the pain I had to see in his eyes, were more than I thought I'd ever have to see. I couldn't answer his questions, I couldn't make the pain go away, and I couldn't even promise him that Logan would be all right. I felt absolutely helpless. That's how I would sum up TTTS: helpless. Each time we thought things would be fine, they weren't. We could never let our guard down for fear that the other shoe would drop.

TUMMERS: Cameron continued to struggle with weight. For many months, he was on fortified breast milk as well as reflux medication. (We had many scary episodes of choking, thanks to reflux). At around 6 months, things changed at last, and he quickly made it onto the growth chart! At a year, he was finally on par for his gestational age.

He has received physio for many months and appears to be catching up to his gestational age group. He has the most relaxed and happy personality, and is a joy to be around. People stop us everywhere to ask us about him; it seems he attracts a lot of attention.

We are open and honest with everyone, especially Cameron and his older brothers, about our little angel, Cole. We say "hi" and pray each day for Cole.

Cameron is fascinated with his reflection in the mirror. I often wonder if this is his way of playing with his brother. He cannot handle being alone, unless he's asleep or going to bed. I am quite certain he misses Cole very much, just like his Mommy does!

LIGHT: We made it out with both of our children. They're completely healthy kids; their weight difference is the only abnormality (if you can even call it that). Once they were both home from the NICU, we never slept. We had to feed them fortified Formula every 3 hours, even in the middle of the night. We don't remember the first three months very well.

MORGAN: I am so proud to say I have a survivor. He is healthy, very active, and not at all disabled. When we came home from the hospital, we were greeted by our family. We all felt so relieved and lucky to have a healthy baby. I had planned to choose a daycare center, but ultimately decided to stay home with him.

HOPE: I am blessed to have two healthy survivors. Jorja had a lot of growth problems and trouble putting on weight, but that is really all. At the age of 6, she is the weight of a full grown 2 year old, but that doesn't stop her. Both girls do well at school, have no major health problems, and are bright, happy and energetic girls.

The day Chloe came home from hospital was very sad. I felt like I was leaving a huge part of me behind. I cried most of the trip home, but inside I tried hard to remember to celebrate taking one of my baby girls home. Jorja's homecoming was quite different. We called every morning to see how she was and to check her weight gain. Jorja would only be allowed to come home when she had reached just over 4 lbs. We knew that could be any day. I rang one of her regular nurses and, like always, my first question was, "Has she been weighed and what is her weight?" That day, the nurse's voice dropped as she said, "Oh chook, I'm sorry; she weighs 4lb 5oz." My face dropped and I just shook my head at David. Then, what she said registered with me. I burst into tears and told David she was coming home. The nurse cracked up and said, "Get off the phone and hurry up and get here. I am sick of her today; she is all yours." Leaving the hospital this time was different -- I was leaving with both my little girls, safe and sound in the back of the car.

WRIGHT: Julie Anne is our sole survivor. She is loved by so many people, and one of the happiest and most content babies. She needed three brain surgeries to place a VP shunt to manage the Hydrocephalus, and the stroke she suffered when Sarah died left her with some weakness on her left side. Though she is delayed in some areas, in others she is either advanced or right on. Julie Anne receives Occupational and Physical Therapy to help her recover from her stroke, but she always brings joy to everyone she meets.

DILLE: I have a beautiful, strong, loving survivor named Cara Grace. She was born at near full term and has no lasting effects from her TTTS, other than the loss of her twin sister. She may be the happiest baby I have ever seen, always smiling and laughing.

Cara constantly gives me hugs and kisses. I like to think Tessa tells Cara that Mommy needs extras, from her.

It was hard for me when Cara first came home from the hospital. Actually, it was leaving the hospital that was hardest for me. I felt as though I was abandoning Tessa there, and that made me feel guilty. I wanted so desperately to be happy bringing home my new baby girl, but there was just an overwhelming sadness at being unable to bring home both girls. I tried my hardest to focus on being positive for Cara's sake. There were plenty of times that I found myself just enjoying Cara, and that made me happy for the moment.

Personally, I cannot put my survivor, Cara, in daycare. I've always been home with my other children; I want to be the one who raises them full time, and I find it hard to trust other people with my children. I have a more difficult time leaving Cara than my older two. I live in almost constant fear that something else is going to happen to her, especially when I am away. Most people adopt the attitude "bad things won't happen to me or my children", but the worst did happen to me; I lost my child. My world will never be the same.

BRAY: Our survivor, Thomas Oliver Bray, is now a bouncing one year old baby. His weight has caught up and he is doing fantastically. He has been discharged from the preemie clinic, and only sees the health visitor as often as other children his age.

OROSZ: Both my babies survived. We have two strong little fighters. They are gaining weight now and doing well at home. The day they came home was the greatest. I ended up having some baby blues, because when they were in the hospital, I didn't get to do the normal motherly things. Though I was recovering from the c-section, and told not to drive for a week, my husband was working and I needed to be with my boys at the hospital, so I started driving there the day after I got out. I cleaned and drove back and forth to the hospital daily; I didn't have time to think.

We are all doing well now. Blake (recipient) has an ear tag, and needs an ultrasound of his kidneys to look out for trouble. I could never put the kids in day care. It's hard to trust people you don't know with your children.

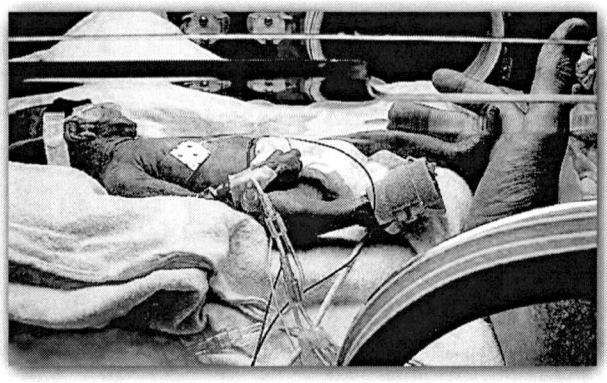

FLETCHER: Allyson is a miracle indeed, but a little smaller than most two year olds. You would never know how she started out. She now weighs over 21 lbs. and is almost 32 inches tall. She talks all the time, and runs and plays with her big brother. She is so loving and sweet, but rotten at the same time - mean enough for her and Abby both. She wears glasses and has had tubes put in, but other than that, nothing really major after NICU. She is a drama queen; they didn't call her the Queen Bee in NICU for nothing, that is for sure. She has a normal life, loved by all who meet her. After she turned a year old, her doctor, Dr. S., wanted to get her into the Tennessee Early Intervention Program , so she wouldn't get too far behind developmentally. After a year in the program, she graduated out. She only had one slight delay, but it wasn't enough to keep her enrolled, which is very unusual for preemie. This is where we met Alice Browder and Kim Ketron, two amazing women.

Ally has been in a daycare. She started a program at one of our area high schools, called Mini-Raiders. It was only a couple of days a week for a few hours. I just wanted to see how she would do, and how it would be if and when I went back to work. She loved the program and met some new friends. One of her Mini-Raider teachers was my mini-raider in high school, and after whom Abbigial Laken was named. Allyson is a special little girl and a ball of energy. She surprises us more and more every day. God is good. We are so thankful to have Austin and Ally here with us, to watch them grow.

DOBBS: I had a long talk with God and asked Him, if He was going to take Emilee, to please let me see her and get to say goodbye. I did not want her to suffer and be in pain. When I was able to see her for the first time, I was only able to hold her for a few seconds because they were afraid she was going to have a stroke if put under too much stress. I held her and kissed her and told her I loved her with all of my heart. Michael and I spent the rest of that day sitting by her incubator, talking to her. The nurses said she was the biggest baby in the NICU, but that she was very sick and we needed to give her body time to heal. We met with the doctors and Social Services later that afternoon, and were told the girls definitely had TTTS. They explained that the TTTS had attacked all of Emilee's organs, but mostly her digestive system. They had put in in a feeding tube, to help her get the nutrients she needed. We were going to have to give her time, let her body recover, realize that her blood was like sand, and be patient to see if it started working on its own. She had yet to have a bowel movement, and would vomit anything she was given. They did an ultrasound on her heart, liver, and kidneys, and said everything looked good. My husband left her, for the first time, to take me home. The phone rang at 4:00 am; she had developed an infection and they were starting a course of antibiotics. It would be another 10 to 15 days before she could come home.

Her bowels caught up and she was able to eat a teaspoon of breast milk every 20 minutes. I never thought I could be so happy about a bowel movement, but it was a happy day.

Five days later, she was transferred to step down. We called the social worker and Dr. M., to see if we could have her sent back to Wheeling, and his care. He agreed that he would handle her case from then on, so she went back, by ambulance. That was another happy day for us; for the first time, we were able to hold her and feed her. She was five days shy of a month old. The commute to Wheeling everyday was a dream come true, and to finally have our little girls back together was a miracle.

Ashlee and Emilee met their sister, Kendra, on January 13, 2006. Ashlee stopped moaning as soon as

she was sleeping beside her sister. They are insepara-
ble, with very few side effects from the TTTS. Ashlee
has hearing loss in her left ear, and acid reflux, so she
has to be checked for low iron every once in a while.
Emilee, on the other hand, has no physical side effects. They have been working with a speech therapist since they came home, which continues two days
a week.

WALLINGTON: We had a very good outcome to our
experience, but I am painfully aware that this is not
everyone's story. For those families that could not
have the surgery, or whose little ones did not make it,
I am truly sorry for their pain. I am sure that these
families would say the same thing to any of the mothers that are struggling with TTTS.

BRUCE: Taylor was born weighing 2.13 lbs. She was
on a ventilator for less than two weeks, but remained
in the NICU for six weeks. She required no surgeries,
only three blood transfusions. Basically, she just
needed to eat and grow, so we were very lucky. She
was released from the NICU on October 25, 2007,
weighing 4.5 lbs. She came home with oxygen for
during feedings, and an apnea monitor. The apnea
monitor was a true pain. The leads had to be posi-
tioned just right or the alarm would sound, which
was the loudest noise I have ever heard -- louder than
being right by a smoke alarm when it goes off. There
were many times when I was awakened in the middle
of the night by the monitor, which meant Taylor had
stopped breathing and her heart rate was decreasing.
It got to the point where I didn't even fall asleep some
nights, because I was too afraid.

After two days, we realized that something wasn't right; the monitor was alarming every 15 minutes or so. We took Taylor to Children's Healthcare of Atlanta at Egleston, where she was readmitted to NICU. After watching her for three days, they determined she had acid reflux, which was the cause of all the alarms. They sent her home with a prescription, and in a few days, her reflux was under control and the monitor quit alarming.

Taylor is growing up beautifully. Her weight and height finally caught up with her age by 2 years old. On the twins' birthday, which is also the day Jordyn died, we go to the cemetery with flowers and balloons. I take pictures of Taylor at Jordyn's grave. When dark falls on the twins' birthday, we release lanterns with messages to Jordyn on them. We also have a small birthday cake with Jordyn's name on it. These rituals may sound abnormal to a person who hasn't lost a child, but we want to make sure that Taylor knows she had an identical twin sister. Recognizing Jordyn has been extremely healing for our whole family. Taylor was 3 months away from her third birthday when she first spoke her sister's name. It sounded sweet coming out of her mouth.

33
What Can a Mother With a TTTS Pregnancy Expect?

Mrs. Jelley was pregnant, with TTTS, while this book
was being created. I thought it would be important
for her to voice her emotions on a current timeline.
She was pregnant with triplets, but only one survived. I asked her to answer some questions, if she
was able.

<u>What do you expect?</u> I hope I can heal. I hope my
baby girl will come home and I
can go on with life without freaking out every day.

<u>What do you expect people to say to you?</u> "I'm sorry"
has to be the best thing for people to say. It kind of
depends on who it is, whether or not I actually want
to be asked anything, but anyone that will acknowledge that they were my children gets my blessing. It
wasn't just a miscarriage, though I can't belittle that
pain either. I feel that I knew my girls. I imagined
their personalities, their smiles, and what I would say
to them when they were older. I am a mother of triplets always, a mother of five. I will struggle whenever
anyone asks me how many kids I have, because I already want to avoid bringing up the disease. It
would be easier to just forget that it happened.

<u>What has been the biggest surprise about your preg-
nancy?</u> No one knew about TTTS.

<u>What do you wish would happen now? Are your
surprised with all of your emotions?</u> I'm very surprised. I know that I still believe in God, but I don't
trust Him right now. I want to, though, and I keep

praying that He will be patient with me. But I prayed almost every day for my girls, and it didn't matter. I believe I won't become bitter, and I hope to soon get over this part. I can be so angry; it just isn't right. I wanted them SO badly. I still want them. I miss them.

Do you have a support group? The most support I have is from Facebook. I've been connected with a lot of women that have one survivor from TTTS and it does help a little; I wish I didn't feel so alone. People drive me crazy, all the time. They say the wrong things. One lady commented on how the meanings of my girls' names were so cool, saying it was perfect that Ellina was the one that made it, since her name is Joy and she will bring joy. I took that to mean, "Good thing you lost the other two." I know she meant well, but I don't want just anybody talking about my babies. I find that right now, I don't want to interact right with anyone I'm not close with.

How is your husband coping? My husband doesn't seem to know how to cope. I worry about him because he won't talk to me. He has gone to see Ellina, but he seems to avoid thinking about it. He doesn't tell me much, but I'm pretty sure he's afraid of getting attached, though he is so attached already.

Do you feel that that you and your husband are communicating well? My husband just doesn't talk much when he's upset. I know sometimes he talks a little more with his friends, but it's just so hard for him. It helps that I have him somewhat figured out, so if he says a couple of things, I know what he's feeling.

What advice is your doctor giving you? My doctor seemed to feel the finality when he discharged me. It was a sad talk. Although he seems to have a hard time talking about the girls, I want to blame him for some of the things that he's said, because he sounds almost hard about it. But somehow, I know that he really does care, and I know he tried his best to save all my girls.

<u>How are you coping with having your daughter in the NICU?</u> Nothing feels right. My baby isn't supposed to be out yet. I should not have to feel torn; I should have her safe in my belly. It's torturous knowing all the things they have to do to her, seeing her picline IVs, when she's so tiny. When I hold her, everything feels right, but it's brief, because when I give her back, I feel like a part of me is gone.

Our girls were named Emmalin Mercy, Ellina Joy, and Ellianna Hope.

34
Our Losses: How Did We Make It?

"When we lose our parents, we are orphans.

When we lose our spouse, we are widows.

But there is no word for a parent who loses a child.

There has never been a word, in any language, to describe the agony of losing our children."

- Author Unknown.

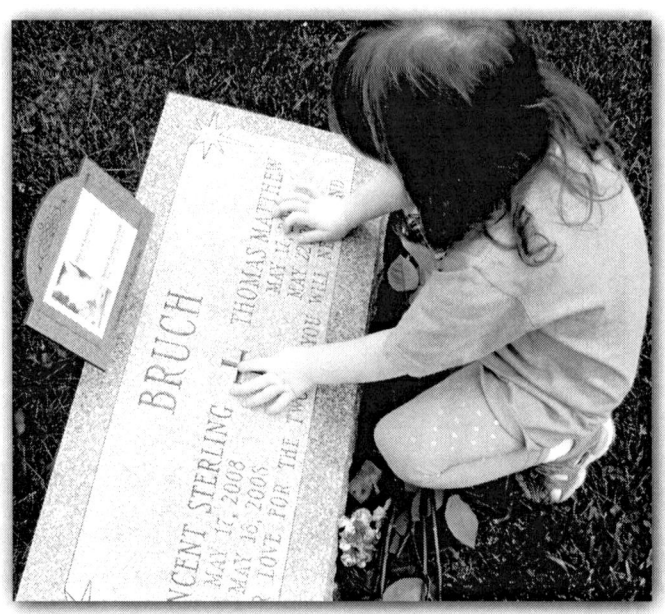

BRUCH: Vincent lived for one day and Thomas lived for five. Vincent died from the shock of being born too early; he was just too small. Thomas put up a great fight. Before Thomas passed, I was in my hospital bed when my sister came in to visit him and me. She looked at me, and said she had a confession to make. When I asked what it was, she said that she hadn't believed me, that she thought TTTS was something that I made up, or that I was being a hypochondriac. But now that she was helping plan a funeral for her godson, she realized that she, herself, couldn't deal with it, and she needed to say she was sorry for not believing me. I quickly said it was ok, but we still had to stay strong.

The week after they passed, I would wake up feeling my belly, and wishing I was still pregnant. It wasn't until seven weeks after the joint funeral that I began to feel the emotional pain of it all. It was like walking in a fog, unsure of where you're going. I saw a therapist, and went to group therapy for neonatal loss. I had to come to grips with the physical and emotional sides of what had happened. Through this, I lost my own identity, struggling with the question "Am I still a mother?" Thank God for Now I Lay Me Down To Sleep Portraits -- they are angels. Their photographer came to my house, picked up some pictures of my sons, perfected them, and put them on a cd for me. It was so great to have touched up pictures of my babies. He didn't even charge me for them.

I have asked family and friends who came to see me at the hospital what went on, since I still can't remember. My dad recalls the day I held Vincent, only hours after he passed. Dad looked at my sister, my mother and me. He describes what he saw as "an air of saint hood". He said, "How we were there, in this horrible situation, just getting each other through it… Erin, it was just an awe-inspiring sight".

My parents took the reins for the service. They had planned it for Vincent, so when Thomas passed in my arms the day before it was to take place, they just added him. Vincent and Thomas are buried together in a blue blanket, I think. To be honest, I can't say for certain, some things are still so cloudy. My family did so much for me that I can never repay them. I mean, what parent plans a funeral service for a grandbaby. I would rather wonder about a future college tuition bill than a headstone bill.

Three weeks after their birthday, I woke up and the pain was too great. I looked at my prescription medication and thought, "If I take them all, I could be with them." Thankfully, my daughter woke up, and I stopped myself. That day I realized I needed help, and began to see a therapist. It was a gut check. My husband came with me at first, to make sure I was in good hands. I saw the therapist for a year and a half after the loss. At first I felt weird, but then I realized it was what I needed, and became fine with it. The therapist put me on medication to ease the stress. Remembering this today, I am just so lost, wondering why none of my doctors ever referred me for counseling.

HADDIGAN: We were headed to the hospital within a couple of hours, when the phone rang. The doctor's voice said, "Riley was a sick baby before, but he is a really sick baby now. You need to get up here as quickly as you can. Do you have someone with you?" This would be a terrible day. When we got there, the

doctor came to tell us that they'd done all they could
for Riley, but we were too late. We never had a
chance to tell him good-bye, to touch him one last
time, to tell him we love him. He was gone. They
brought him to us wrapped in a blanket; he had on a
little white gown and a white hat. The wires and
tubes were gone. He was perfect. We each held him,
wishing that somehow it wasn't real, that it was all
just a horrible nightmare and we'd wake up - please
let us wake up! But this was it, our reality.

We went to see Logan and the nurses rushed to
let us hold him for the first time. As I held him, all I
could think was that I wanted to just leave there with
him, just take him home with me. I couldn't imagine
leaving him there while there was the nightmarish
possibility that he could leave me to be with his
brother.

SLICHTER: The week after was horrible for us. The
first few days I felt like a zombie, walking around my
house. I would feel my stomach, and it was so flat I
would just break down. My husband comforted me
in every way that he knew how. I knew that he was
grieving, too, and that this was hard for him as well,
though sometimes I thought not. I know now that we
all have different ways of grieving. He would go to
work and cry, instead of crying in front of me.

We tried to resume as normal a life as possible.
I got a job, and my husband went back to work.
Things just weren't getting any easier, or happier. We
were often late for work since we were both in severe
states of depression, yet we didn't know it. I often
asked myself, "Why? Why us?" I tried to blame everything and everyone. I wondered, if something we

did had been done differently, would I still have my babies? Nothing in the world really mattered; it was like we had just stopped as the world flew by us. We were sad all the time, just feeling sorry for ourselves and mad at whoever didn't feel the same. We lost some friends and didn't make new ones. We were sent to a counselor, who said that I was fine, and what I was experiencing was normal, but I knew it wasn't. Life was horrible. We had each other, and only each other, so we grew very close, more in love, and still are to this day. We did everything they say to do to help with the grieving process, but nothing seemed to help. We were still heavily grieving the loss of our babies and our life was like that for a year.

DICK: We had their funeral on June 2, 2007, and then had them cremated. Their urn now sits on a shelf my parents made in memory of them. I can't help but think, "Could the doctors have done something to save my babies?" or "Was it really too late?" I know I can't change it now, but the "what ifs" never leave my mind. Do they ever go away, the "what ifs"? Will I ever be able to forgive the doctors? I don't know that they did anything wrong, but I still feel like they should've held to their promise… if they were at least a pound, they would try. My Brookelynn passed away beforehand, but my Jazmen was alive. I held her and felt her chest rise and fall with each breath. I felt her touch. She was a pound and she was born alive and they could do NOTHING. Was she too far gone? I don't know, but I can't get over the "what ifs".

CADLE: January12, 2006, I was induced, and told

"these things happen." Because it was before 20 weeks, they considered it a miscarriage. Ronnie, my dad, my step mom, and I were there for a few hours, waiting to see if I was going to deliver. My dad and step mom left after the nurse said it was going to be a long time. My sisters, mom, and mother-in-law were all on their way, so that was okay. Two of my sisters, Lynda and Beth, got there just in time. I had dilated to 4cm and was ready to push. I remember looking up at my sister, Lynda, shaking my head "no," and saying I did not want to have them. I pushed, and we had three precious little boys: Talin Matthew Cadle (9oz., 13cm long), Blain Matthew Cadle (7oz., 11cm long), and Drake Matthew Cadle (3oz., 6cm long).

They had no heartbeats. Nothing I was told had been true! The staff did not clean them up. My doctors and other medical personnel sucked! Sorry for being so blunt, but I was mistreated and over-looked. No one truly cared about my boys and me. The nurses took some lousy pictures and gave me three of everything, but other than that they were use-less.

When the nurse came and said, "Do you want to hold them?" I said no. She offered to wash them off and wrap them up, if I wanted to see them, but I couldn't. I had no idea what to say or what to do. I was lost.

My family was all there the next day. My mom, oldest sister, Amanda, and my mother-in-law went in to see them and took a few pictures, but nothing was like it should have been. I should have held them, looked at them, taken pictures of them, but I did not, and I am having trouble healing because of that horrible choice. They were my children; I should have done what every mother does when she has her babies. It has been a few years and I have a hard time getting through. I still struggle, but it's not as devastating.

MORGAN: I am different than a lot of people. I can't seem to grieve like others. Growing up, my dad was true blue-collar and always told me that crying never really helps anything. Through the years, I realized that he was right. He was the first person I wanted to talk to.

Emilee was at my mom's house. Mom and my nanny live next door to each other, so whenever things happen, it's my mom's job to watch Emilee. I didn't call my mother at 3:30am even though I wanted to, because I knew she would come when Emilee got up. Everything kind of settled down at the hospital. After my mom came, I called my dad. When I did, he asked me what I was going to do next. To this day, that question stands as the most important question of my life. My answer was: to take care of Emilee and love her even more than before. After all, she needed me; she was and still is my child. The boys were in Heaven, with my recently passed grandfather.

I didn't shed any tears until I got in our truck to go home. I couldn't grasp reality. Why would such a thing happen to us and our innocent baby boys? I did cry for a while, and even now my husband and I can't really talk about it, or maybe we just don't. I tend to place things in my head and let them be. My mom tells me that my head is like an old fashioned roll-top desk, the kind with all the filing drawers. She tells me that when something bad happens, instead of it really affecting the outside of me, I file it away in one of my many "drawers," which take a lot for me to open back up. I guess that is my survival mechanism.

We had a graveside service that my nanny paid for. We had some sort of discount, as we had just buried my grandfather the same year. We did have a decent turn out, even though it was very hot outside. My mom was my strength through it all, but my mother-in-law was the thorn in my side. She made everything about her, which didn't help anything at all. She acted like she was the one who had to endure it all, and was no help with any of our emotions. She didn't talk to me in the hospital; instead, she showed off. She was the one person that made the situation worse for me.

A very close friend of the family officiated the ceremony. It was so touching. We didn't want to let the boys go, and just stared at the box where they lay. My mom had made them shirts to wear, and the funeral home gave them bears to be buried with. To bury your children, looking at a box with them inside… no words can describe the situation. I went back to church, only to be approached by a church member who informed me that her daughter was pregnant. I just wanted to get up and leave; it was hard to go back after that. I mean, I had just been through a very traumatic experience in my life. Please don't come up to me with stuff like that; think of my feelings, for once.

I did find a lot of comfort in an online group called L.A.M.B.S. The women on there really helped, along with another group called HANDS, which found me. One day, I got this mysterious envelope in the mail with a "life certificate" enclosed. I don't know how they found me, or got my information, but it was so nice. The lady molds clay to look and feel like your lost babies. I've heard it really helps some people.

TUMMERS: The absolute worst part of losing Cole was telling his older brothers that we wouldn't be bringing two babies home from the hospital after all. It was the most difficult discussion I've ever had to have. We *tried* to read "We Were Gonna Have a Baby, But We Had an Angel Instead." I didn't tell anyone else, I let Geoff do it. I posted a note on Facebook and sat back to let people come to me.

The first three weeks after Cole died were awful. It was Christmas, and my other kids needed me, so I had no choice but to function. Each time I saw someone new, I'd start to cry. The worst time of day was morning, before the boys woke up. I'd lie there and cry and wonder how I'd ever get by. I spent a lot of time on the computer; the TTTS Foundation and Fetal Hope kept me going. I was so fearful, all of the time, that I'd lose Cameron, too. I was also stressed about delivery and meeting them both. After my water broke at 26 weeks and we were sure that Cameron was going to be born, reality set in. I needed to get my head in a better place, because this might all happen right away.

Thank God it didn't. In the hospital, I was allowed to be alone with my thoughts and feelings, with no interruptions from my loving kids or hubby. I was able to think, to process, and to grieve, somewhat. Things also became very clinical; my pregnancy seemed to be treated as if I was expecting a

singleton, and that hurt. I got a social worker in-
volved right away, to help everyone understand my
feelings, including me. Things seemed okay, and I
was coping, until the delivery date was set. Then I
was such a mess and cried every day. I knew I
wanted to hold Cole, wrapped in the matching blankets, but I didn't know if I wanted to see him. I did
want to hold them together, one last time. Unfortunately, when the day arrived, those directions seemed
to have gotten lost with the staff.

My midwife was able to be with me throughout the C-section. She stayed with Cole, and helped
to wash and dress him. She tried to take his foot-
prints and handprints, but they didn't turn out very
well. Nor did the picture she took of him, but perhaps that is a blessing. She brought him to me as I
was still being closed up, but I knew I couldn't do it
then. When I got to recovery, she brought him to me
again. She told me he was perfect, laid him on my
chest, and took the blanket from his tiny body. He
had a little hat on, and wore a small knitted outfit that
wasn't really on him, just around him. My first
thought, though, wasn't how perfect he was. It pains
me to say this, but I never thought that. I was fairly
disturbed by his face. He had been gone for 11 weeks,
so his skin and features were breaking down. I was
just so damned emotional that I couldn't bond with
my baby. I wanted to look at him, I wanted to touch
his skin, but I couldn't bring myself to do it and I hate
that now.

My husband and parents joined me and we
cried and cried. No one else wanted to look at Cole,
but everyone wanted to hold him. It was by far the
hardest few moments of my life. My heart was break-

ing, my arms were aching, and I just felt so terribly alone. After everyone had some time with him, the nurses took him back to the warm room. We knew we would need to see him again, but were just feeling too emotional, and overwhelmed with all those people around. Then, I finally got to see Cameron. Looking back now, I realize how perfectly odd it was to see the baby I hadn't worried about for 11 weeks first. I knew Cole was safe in God's hands, but Cameron wasn't, yet I hadn't thought of him since Cole had been placed in my arms.

Later that night, the nurse came to our room asking if we wished to see Cole again. He was brought to us in a tiny bassinette, and hadn't been covered up. I knew my husband couldn't handle seeing his face, so I asked the porter to cover him up again, though I really wanted to spend time looking at him. We spent about half an hour with him, telling him about his brothers, our family, and our dreams for him. My husband had such a tough time letting him go, and I guess in our hearts, we never will.

We had decided, weeks earlier, that we would have him cremated. We wanted to plant a memory garden and put his ashes there. In time though, we decided this wasn't the best plan, as the garden then became a sacred place we'd never want to be anything but perfect, and what happened if we ever moved? We decided to plant the garden at our home, and have our friends place stones and plants there, in his memory. My parents will buy their plots, and later his ashes will be buried there. To do the garden, we needed to postpone our service until it was warm enough to plant, too. We wanted to have Cameron baptized at the same time but for a few good reasons, our church wouldn't allow this. No one seemed to get that we needed to honor them together.

On May 31st , we finally had our boys welcomed into God's family, and said goodbye to our angel. It was a very emotional service, filled with music and scripture. My husband and I both spoke to about fifty mourners. We then had Cameron dedicated, and everyone came to our backyard to place tributes in Cole's garden. Our friend, a minister and the mom of 25.5 week fraternal twin girls, dedicated and blessed it.

CHRISTMAN-SCHARER: At 5:45 Tuesday morning, while getting ready to go, we got a call telling Karl that Karlyn was having problems and we should get there ASAP. They told him they had to do CPR; a lot of things had happened throughout the night. I was in the shower, and he didn't tell me any of this right away, since he didn't want to worry me. I wish he had at least told me to get my mom there ASAP, but instead we woke the kids early, got them dressed, and took them to daycare before we were on our way. We arrived at St. Christopher's around 9 am, about three hours after they called. She was already gone. Karl saw her doctor in the lobby; he took us to a room and started talking. I thought he was reporting her status before we went to see her, but no. He told us everything about her condition, and what they had done for her. He said they made a valiant effort to save her, but that at 7:10 am, she passed away. They tried to call our cell phones, but since there was no reception where we were, we never got the call. I think that was a blessing, because it would have been horrible to find out over the phone. Karl and I sat there, crying. I couldn't believe it. What a horrible mom I was, to put my other children and resting ahead of going to see my sick daughter. She must hate me. I should have gone Monday night. I thought that maybe if I had, she would have made it.

They took us to our little angel, Karlyn. A nurse there said she had never left her side. They handed us two little ceramic squares with hearts on them, and told us they caught her last two heartbeats. We were given all the blankets, hats and things that were hers. Then, they brought her in and let us hold her. They took some pictures of her, and we took some also. We only had two pictures of her alive; the rest were taken after she passed away. She was all wrapped up, and I opened her blankets and just looked at her. She was perfect; all her parts were there. Her ears weren't fully formed because she was actually about a 24 week baby, and she was bruised, but that didn't stop me from holding and kissing her. I didn't want to leave her. I wanted her back in my belly, which was the last time I knew she was really ok. We might have stayed until 7 that night, but decided we couldn't sit there that long. We had lost one daughter; we needed to go to the other, and make sure she was ok. I called my mom and told her. She and dad wanted to see Karlyn, but it was too painful for Karl and me to sit there another three hours, waiting for them. I needed to focus on Kylie and make sure she was ok.

I had this weird thought on the way home; I wished we could have brought Karlyn home with us instead of leaving her there. She needed me. I could take her to the funeral home. I know, what a thought! We called our parents, who helped us with the other kids, and with arranging the funeral for Karlyn. Let

me say, burying your child is the hardest thing anyone could ever do! It is heartbreaking. Karl and I
seemed to breeze through all of the planning on auto-
pilot. We were dazed and shocked.

We met my family at the hospital, and took my
parents, my youngest brother, and his wife in to see
Kylie. I took Karlyn's things in with me, too. Kylie
was doing well. (Actually, after Karlyn died, Kylie
improved daily.) That day, they let us touch and hold
her, which was comforting. I think that when Karlyn
died, she gave Kylie the energy to get stronger, so she
could come home with us. I feel Karlyn is a part of
Kylie. She lives through her.

We headed home then, and got the boys from
daycare. We told Tyler and Alex that Karlyn died.
Tyler, only 8, started crying. Alex was 6 and didn't
cry. I don't think it hit him right away. Reid, of
course, was too young to understand at only one. Tyler and Alex were upset, and kept saying, "We didn't
get to meet her or hold her!" I felt so badly for them.
My heart was breaking for my little girl and breaking
for my boys at the same time. I had to be strong for
them, so I explained that she was too sick. They were
worried about Kylie, so I told them she was doing
fine. We took them to see her that night.

Karlyn's funeral took place on 6/30/06, seven
days after she was born. Karl and I were still in
shock. We were going to limit the open casket to immediate family, because she was bruised, but when
we saw her at the funeral home, she looked like she
did when she was born, very white. We decided to
have an open casket for everyone. This was the one
and only time they would see my beautiful identical

twin daughter, Karlyn. Almost all of my family and friends were there, even my team from work. Karl's parents and three members of his family were there, but no one from work. I felt so bad for him. Karl has a big family; when the majority of them decided not to come, it hurt us very badly. Karl's mother told us not to be mad. I wanted to ask her, "How would you feel if they didn't show up when your daughter died? Would you be ok with it?" We didn't cry a lot that day, except during her eulogy, and when we had to leave her at the cemetery. Alex finally cried at the cemetery. I think the finality hit him.

We had a big party for Karlyn and Kylie's first birthday and also for Reid, who turned two in June. We invited Karl's family again and this time, they all showed up, but only because an aunt told them how rude they were for not going to the funeral and supporting us. Karl's mom always tries to get us to go to their children's events, but I have a hard time doing anything with his side of the family. They weren't there for us, so why should I care about them? I know that sounds harsh, but when my daughter died, my life and attitude changed. Life is short, but I cannot forgive his family for not being there. They have no excuse for not showing up.

MORGAN: I still don't feel I have recovered from the loss. I cried a lot, at home by myself, while my husband was at work. I never had a service for my son, which I regret. I was told by my doctors and family that he had been in my tummy for so long, he had basically "dissolved" into my system. There wasn't much left of him.

BENNER: I had decided to make sure to hold them on the day we found out we had TTTS. We took pictures, made a video, and told them how much we loved them. I will never forget the time I spent with them.

After I delivered the boys, they had to remove the placenta. I didn't know that after you are in labor, you must push it out. I wasn't that far along and couldn't; it was still attached to the wall of my uterus. I began to get sick, and started shaking convulsively. My blood pressure rose, and I had a very high temperature. I wanted to sleep, but I had nurses prodding and picking at me. They brought a wheelchair and took me to surgery. The room had bright lights; I sat on the table and was given a spinal tap. Everything got blurry and I couldn't feel anything from my waist down. They performed a D and C to remove the placenta. After the surgery I was in recovery for about four hours. The boys were still in my room. I wanted to wake up and find it was all a dream. A nurse came in to check on me, clean me up, and put socks on my feet. I remember her nice gestures. All the nurses were nice, probably because of the situation. But I think that's what I needed.

After recovery, we spent time with the boys, took more pictures, and said we loved them, but never said goodbye. I remember that they were so cold, and I felt so bad because there wasn't anything I could do.

WRIGHT: We had a small memorial service and burial for our Sarah. Being able to go "visit" my little girl has been helpful in the grieving process. I believe I am still "getting through" the loss of my daughter. Some days are better than others. I have learned to let myself cry whenever I feel the need and to not hold back. I have found quite a few other TTTS mommies, and talking with them has been a huge help. Knowing that there are other moms who have been through the same thing is invaluable. When I start to get down about the loss of my baby girl, I try to focus on my surviving daughter and be thankful that Sarah is in a better place. I know I'll see her again one day.

DILLE: Though nothing has really gotten me through the loss of my baby, Tessa, if I had to pick something, it would be my other children, including Cara. Being a Mom is very important to me. I have always put my children first; they are my world. Being there for them is more important than anything else in life. There have been times since our loss that I just wanted everything to be over, so the pain would end. In those times, I thought of my children, and how much they needed me to be strong for them.

The thought of finally meeting my survivor, Cara, also helped me get through the loss of Tessa. Since I lost Tessa right after the surgery at 20 weeks, and carried Cara almost to term, I still had almost half of my pregnancy to go. It was so hard to know that I was still carrying two babies, but would only be bringing one home. I so looked forward to the day when I could finally have my survivor in my arms.

Another thing that helped me through the remainder of my pregnancy, and up until now, is the group of TTTS Moms that I've met online. I don't know if I could make it without the support of these Moms, who truly know what I am going through. Other people can try and sympathize with the situation, but only Moms who have experienced the same thing can truly understand.

My husband and I chose to have a funeral for Tessa. I felt she needed to be recognized as a person, and my daughter, whom I loved. She had a beautiful, tiny casket, which my mom carried to and from the altar. We had lovely flowers arranged to put next to her. While the day did give us some closure after so many months, it was even more painful than the day that Tessa died. My son, who was 7 at the time, was very emotional throughout the entire service, but tried to hide it. I told him over and over that it was okay for him to be sad and to cry. Cara was a perfect baby, sleeping and snuggling with me during the funeral.

My husband and I chose to have Tessa cremated. Never in a million years would I think that this was something I would ever do, but I felt like I needed to have a part of her with me always. I have a special teardrop necklace with some of her ashes in it. I don't wear it every day, but I do wear it when I'm feeling especially upset or want to be close to her. Whenever I wear it, Cara holds it in her hand. I like to think that she knows she's holding a part of her twin sister. Tessa was buried and we had a beautiful headstone made for her. It says, "Always loved, never forgotten."

BRAY: Since losing Oliver and bringing Thomas home, I have become a very over protective mummy. Thomas is now one, and still in his cot in our bedroom. I check on both children around fifteen times throughout the night. I am now a very anxious person, as a result of TTTS.

Losing Oliver is, without a doubt, the hardest thing I have ever had to go through in my life. It's been just over a year since we lost him, and I still visit his grave every day. I cry a lot and miss him terribly, but I have come to terms with things; I have accepted that Oliver is not here and that I will never see my twins grow together, but every day, I will always see Oliver in the face of his identical twin brother. I am lucky; I will be able to see what my little angel would have looked like as he grew.

The fact that I got to take a baby home from hospital has helped more than I realized. I was not left with empty arms. I have the love of two other children to help me through, along with fantastic friends and family who sit and listen to me, who help me with my grief, and keep Oliver's memory alive.

FLETCHER: Abbigial Laken was gone too quickly, but what an impact she left on us. She saved her sister's life - she is a hero, as are all of my children. When we found out that Abby had passed, we lost a piece of us, a light went out in us. I think it is something as a parent you never get over. You are always wondering what they would have been like, but you have to keep your faith and trust in God that he took them for a reason , and one day you will be with them again. I don't think you move on. You just go numb and go on living. You have no choice. As a couple, you have to stay strong for one another and for your kids. I guess what got me through the loss of Abby was God, Scott, Austin, Ally, my family, and friends. I am blessed to have such great people in my life, but Abby is always on my mind. Everything plays like a movie in my head, nonstop. I have my dark days and I have my good days, but I have to get up for Austin and Ally. They are my reason for going on. They bring sunshine to my life when it is raining. Everywhere I go, everywhere I turn, there is always something to remind me of Abby. It is the hardest thing I have ever been through in my life. People told me how strong I was, but I just put up my front. I may seem strong, but I am falling apart on the inside. I think, I will never get to have that moment with Abby, but then I think of her in heaven. No pain, no heartache, no tears. I want her here with me so much, but how could I take her away from the peace of heaven?

Have I been angry? In my darkest moments, yes. Have I asked why? In my darkest moments, yes. The grieving process is a long and hard one, with so many emotions you don't want to endure. I just take it one day at a time, and talk to Abby all of the time.

We had a beautiful service with gorgeous flowers, preaching and singing. "Sheltered in the Arms of God" is where Abby is - that song was sung at her funeral, by Louise Gibson. Brother Johnny Gibson preached, and I remember telling him not to tell her goodbye, but to tell her, "Goodnight Abby; we will see you in the morning." I remember my brother,

Mikey, and Scott's brother, Tim, carrying her little casket. It was so tiny, white with beautiful pink flowers on top. When I turned to watch them bring her into the mausoleum, I thought, are all these people here for Abby? There wasn't anywhere left to sit or stand inside. People stood outside the door. It was amazing. We were so touched to know that so many people cared. It was so hard to know that my baby was in that tiny casket. I can still close my eyes and see it. I don't think there was a dry eye there. People came to hug us at the end, telling me how strong I was, and how I had such faith. I didn't understand how people could see me like that. I am just TJ.

After Brother Johnny preached, I thought, if something good can come out of this, I'll know Abby wasn't taken for nothing. If someone could grow closer to the Lord, or even get saved, that was part of the plan God had for her.

After everyone left, Scott and I stayed until they put her in the ground. After they were done, we had our moment together, as her parents. On the way home, we promised each other that we would still take care of her grave if something was to happen to one of us. No parent should have to have this conversation, but it was our reality. This was what TTTS had done to us.

JELLEY: Cody flew home for good, but it was bittersweet. I will forever miss my two little girls, Emmalin Mercy and Ellianna Hope, but I will thank God that He has given me Ellina.

Our plan had been to hold our babies together, when Cody got back, but when the time came, he couldn't do it. He looked at the pictures, and cried. It was even hard for him to see Ellina.

The next night, I took my friend with me to see the girls. I held them and talked to them. I can still smell them, and see their faces. That night, I couldn't sleep. I ended up sitting next to Ellina's bed, crying. The sweet nurse let me change her diaper and take her temperature. I think that's what got me through that night. I always wonder," if we had just caught it", or, "if I had just done one thing differently…" I go to the NICU and I get angry; there are supposed to be three little cribs for my babies', not just one. I'm supposed to feel torn, but by three live babies, not between a memorial and a baby. It doesn't matter how many people say I did everything right, I still blame myself. I was responsible for them, and I lost them. Why can others carry triplets and I couldn't? It just isn't right, and I wonder what's wrong with me. I have good times, and bad times, when I get so angry. I wonder if throwing a fit would help get rid of the hurt and anger, but I have yet to try it and see. My husband is sad, too, but I can see why we don't talk much about it. If he can be happy for even 5 minutes, I don't want to ruin it for him, drag him down.

BRUCE: We had a graveside service and buried Jordyn on September 18, 2007. It didn't feel real, until I went home and began to take down one of the two cribs. I realized early on that my family and friends love me very much, but have no clue what I go through on a daily basis. My "normal" is no longer the same as their "normal". My "normal" consists of tears at the sight of twins, visits to the cemetery, and a constant feeling of being incomplete. Through the internet, I found other TTTS mothers. We've created an unbreakable bond, even though we've never met.

35
Dealing With Others

BRUCH: By now, I expect people won't know what to say to me. A person does not usually deal with this every day. I have a "jewel kids" necklace, with one charm for each of my children. I will always hate seeing the "deer in the headlights look" every time someone asks, "How many children do you have?" It will drive you to scream.

I have also realized that I live in a new "normal". My life has changed, and I have to understand that. For the most part, I have, but I still wish I had them. Others don't get that, they see me and think, "She's crazy." I'm not; I just miss them, and that is ok.

HADDIGAN: I returned to work part-time while Logan was in the NICU. Most people didn't know what to say, so they said nothing. Some people said all the wrong things. I have since told people that I love to talk about Riley. I love to hear his name. It may make me cry, but it also makes me smile. He's my son, and always will be. The fact that he was only here for four days doesn't make his life any less important. We spent 6 months fighting for him and Logan. We love him and miss him more than I could have ever imagined. Not a day, not an hour, goes by that I don't think of him. I have a charm with his handprint; I kiss it and it makes me feel close to him. I talk to him every day -- somehow it helps me. We plan to send off helium lanterns, with messages to Riley from each of us, on his angel day.

Mother's Day was harder than I expected. I planted forget-me-nots, by myself in the rain. I thought it would make me feel better, but it was painful. I felt like my heart had been ripped out. Some days it seems like he was just here, but others it seems like a hundred years ago that I touched him, felt him in my tummy, saw his perfect little face.

SLICHTER: Dealing with others was hard for me. Many were sympathetic, but a lot of people didn't really know how to react around me. They walked on pins and needles, worried they would say the wrong thing. Many did; they would tell me, "I'm sorry, but don't worry, you're young and you can have more." It was that statement that I absolutely hated. I know I can have more, but I wanted them. I know that many people don't know what to say, and only speak out of the goodness of their heart, but sometimes I was still offended. I was hard for me to look at people who were pregnant or had new babies. I felt very alone, like no one knew what I was going through, and they didn't. No one knows the pain of losing a child until they have been through it.

People who don't know what happened ask me, "When are you going to have children?" so I tell them the story of my boys. I can tell that they are sorry they asked. I love to talk about my babies, but many change the subject quickly. They are my children and I am their mother. What mother doesn't like to talk about her babies? Though mine are not here with me, I love them and think about them every single day of my life.

MARTIN: I still stumble on the children count. A lot

of people look at you weirdly, but to me, I have two girls and two boys (we had a baby girl in September, 2008). Our children's names all start with "E's": Emilee, Ethan, Evan, Ella.

I'm not ashamed to tell anyone. When people ask, I tell them, and they are usually so nice and caring about it. I don't go around telling everyone, even though inside I'm screaming it.

DICK: In the beginning, it was very hard for me to deal with others. Everyone wanted to tell me they were sorry about my loss and how they knew how it felt. But none of them had held their daughter as she took her last breath. None of them had watched their child born into this world sleeping. To me, they knew nothing of what was going on. Though I knew they just wanted to be supportive, I shoved many of them away. Sometimes, I didn't even know if my husband was grieving. He never wanted to talk about them. But as time went on, I realized that he was just as emotional about it as I was, he just handled it in a different way. I guess I felt like no one understood. I had carried these girls for 6 months. I felt their every move, every kick, every tumble, and now they were gone. But as time went by, it became easier to talk about them. The problem was, by then, it seemed like everyone had forgotten. Just because they weren't "here" anymore, everyone moved on. I felt alone again. Then, after a LONG talk with my husband, I realized everyone had stopped bringing them up because they saw how much it hurt me. I also realized I needed to talk about them, to write about them, to speak to them, to celebrate their lives, and not just mourn their deaths.

<u>TUMMERS:</u> For the most part, I don't know how to deal with others. I try to be open and honest about how I feel, which I think puts people off, but I really don't care. I'll never "get over" the loss of my son. I'll never accept that "at least I have one," but I will cope will my loss, and live with the hope that I will see my son again, in Heaven

<u>CHRISTMAN-SCHARER:</u> Dealing with other people after the loss was hard. There were a lot of people saying, "Well at least you have one", or, "You should feel blessed to have your other four". I felt blessed, but I wanted all five of my children here with me.

It was difficult going back to work. There, a lot of people did not know that Karlyn passed away. They asked how "they" were, and when I told them she died after four days, they didn't know what to say. It felt like a lot of people avoided me.

There are several people from work, and friends, who listened to me talk about her and still do now. They know who they are, and I love them for it. They may not understand how it feels to lose a child, but they are always there when I feel the need to talk about her. There are also people who act as if she never existed. That bothers me. They say things about my four kids, but I don't have four kids, I have five. I would love them to acknowledge that, but we cannot change them. We can just move on and not let it bother us.

MORGAN: The hardest part is being asked how many children I have. I immediately want to say I have two babies, but if I did, I would be asked where the other baby is and have to go into detail about what happened. I have told people I have a child in heaven, which often makes them feel uncomfortable or sad for me. When I'm feeling my strongest, I do tell them about TTTS. What else can I do? It's the truth.

I have learned over the past three years that when I have keepsakes of the baby or pictures of my ultrasounds around the house, I get very depressed. I do not want my son to see his mother in a weakened state all the time, and it's not healthy for me to be crying for hours each day. My husband and I feel it's best for our family to keep our child in our memories and hearts. Thankfully, we haven't endured any disrespect for how we are grieving. We are very blessed to have such wonderful friends and family.

BENNER: I always refer to them as "our boys" when I tell people about them. I just stay strong and tell them what I had, and some of what we went through.

The first Christmas was hard. We received ornaments, and a picture frame with the meanings of their names, from my in-laws. On their first birthday, we went back to California and spent a day at the beach. I thought about them the entire time. We wrote their names in the sand. My brother in law gave us cards for their second birthday.

I wish people would see that my way of grieving is just that, my way. They need to accept that, and help me heal in the way that is best for me. For one whole year, people would come up and ask how they

264 | Forever Linked

were doing. I would have to explain to them what had happened. No one was disrespectful about it. We were very fortunate.

WRIGHT: Every time the opportunity arises, I talk about Sarah. Julie Anne's neurological problems would not have happened had Sarah not died, so I find myself telling everyone about my miracle baby and my angel baby in Heaven. Our older children often ask to visit Sarah's grave. They enjoy picking out flowers, stuffed animals, balloons, etc. to take to the grave. They frequently talk about Sarah. My oldest daughter even drew a picture of Sarah with angel wings, lying in a golden crib in Heaven -- how she imagined Sarah was being cared for.

Most people I come in contact with are been very sympathetic and kind in regard to my twins. When Sarah first died, though, a few told me, "At least you still have one left," or, "Well, you could always have another one". It appeared as though Sarah's life didn't matter because she had a twin.

DILLE: Most everyone that we know found out about our loss by word of mouth, so we often didn't have to explain what happened. However, I often find myself in conversations with people about my twin girls. I'm not sure how it comes up, but I do tell people that Cara is a twin, and that I lost her identical twin at 20 weeks, after having a surgery to save them both. I don't go in to much detail about the disease with most people, but I do tell them that TTTS caused our loss.

We definitely keep Tessa a part of our family, and we always will. We bring her flowers, and blow kisses up into the sky to her all the time. I try and talk about her as much as possible without confusing my 3 year old. Our family visits her grave frequently, especially on holidays or anniversaries. We want her to be remembered forever.

I sometimes feel that others should be more respectful of my grieving process. I have actually lost friends over this. Some think that I should be over it by now, or that I should be back to "my regular old self" already. They just don't understand that I will never be the same person I used to be. Losing a child has completely changed me. Most people are quite understanding and empathetic, though. I think people just don't know what to say, so sometimes the wrong thing comes out. They need to understand that just listening to a grieving parent, and telling them that they are sorry, is about the best thing they can do.

In dealing with other people regarding the loss, my biggest shock is that they think because Tessa was not born alive, I did not really lose a child. One acquaintance spoke about a friend of hers who had lost a 6 month old to SIDS. I told her to tell the family how sorry I was, and that losing a child is the worst thing any parent could go through. She responded by saying, "Well I guess yours was a loss, too." Her response was very upsetting.

Another shock is how many people think I am "lucky" because I still have one of my babies. While I am grateful that I do have a survivor, I don't feel lucky to have lost a baby. That's like telling a parent of two children of different ages that it was lucky only one of them died in a car crash, because they got to keep the other one.

After Tessa passed away, people asked me if I had to continue to carry my dead baby until it was time to deliver Cara. I know that most people who asked were probably just curious, but I think they could have researched it, rather than speak to me in that way.

BRAY: Oliver is a very important part of my family. We celebrate his very short life with balloons and a candle, and I involve my earth children as much as I can. I will always tell William and Thomas about Oliver's journey. Thomas is still too young to understand, but William often sends kisses to heaven, and takes flowers to his baby brother's special garden.

FLETCHER: I have found the hardest thing is being asked, "How many kids do you have?" I always answer, "Two angels here, and one waiting on me in heaven." I don't know how else to say it. I have a hard time dealing with people in general, so I want to stay in my house all the time. That way, I don't have to deal with things. Some days, I can talk about it and others, I don't want to. I don't want anyone's pity and I don't want anyone to feel sorry for me. It is something I had to go through along my journey to become who I am today - more guarded, outspoken and not who I once was.

Some people speak before they think. Those are the people that are hard to deal with. I hate hearing, "You are so blessed to have Austin and Ally with you." I know I am, but I have another child that I will not let be forgotten. I remember someone sent a birthday card that said, "Don't think about the things you lost this year". I thought, "Did they not read that before they sent it? That is the one thing I think about all the time!" I am just not going to put Abby's memory away on a shelf and never speak of her again. She is my daughter, too, just as Austin is my son, and Ally is my daughter.

Austin talks about Abby and even cries with me. He says, "I miss my sissy." He has been my little rock. Ally will say her name and point up when you ask her where Abby is. When my kids get older, I will tell them everything that happened, all about TTTS, and let them read this book. How can I forget about all of this, when it is a big part of who our family is? Our lives were changed by the words "Twin to twin transfusion syndrome" and will never be the same. I will always have a piece of Abby here with me through Ally. They say a twin bond is never broken, even in death.

I have grown closer to God through all of this. He is my rock and my salvation.

BRUCE: Sometimes I feel like people have to deal with me, and not the other way around. I love talking about Jordyn, although some individuals look at me strangely when I do open up about her. It's very healing just to talk about her, and hear her name. Her life was just as important as anyone else's, even though that life was short.

36
Suggestions from the moms to others

Here are some things to know when speaking to a mom coping with the loss of a child. I don't know who first wrote them, but many moms have been adding to this list over time.

From the perspective of a mother who has lost a child:

1. I wish my child (children) hadn't died. I wish I had him/her/them back.

2. I wish you wouldn't be afraid to speak my child's (children's) name. My child (children) lived and they were very important to me. I need to hear that they were important to you also.

3. If I cry and get emotional when you talk about my child (children), I wish you knew that it isn't because you have hurt me. My child's (children's) death is the cause of my tears. You have talked about my child (children), and you have allowed me to share my grief. I thank you for both.

4. I wish you wouldn't "kill" my child (children) again by removing their pictures, artwork, or other remembrances from your home or work place.

5. Being a bereaved parent is not contagious, so I wish you wouldn't shy away from me. I need you now more than ever.

6. I need diversions, so I do want to hear about you; but I also want you to hear about me. I might be sad and I might cry, but I wish you

would let me talk about my child (children), my favorite topic of the day.

7. I know that you think of and pray for me often. I also know that my child's (children's) death pains you, too. I wish you would let me know those things through a phone call, a card or note, or a real big hug.

8. I wish you wouldn't expect my grief to be over in six months. These first months are traumatic for me, but I wish you could understand that my grief will never be over. I will suffer the death of my child (children) until the day I die.

9. I am working very hard in my recovery, but I wish you could understand that I will never fully recover. I will always miss my child (children), and I will always grieve that they are dead.

10. I wish you wouldn't expect me "not to think about it" or to "be happy." Neither will happen for a very long time, so don't frustrate yourself.

11. I don't want to have a "pity party," but I do wish you would let me grieve. I must hurt before I can heal.

12. I wish you understood how my life has shattered. I know it is miserable for you to be around me when I'm feeling miserable. Please be as patient with me as I am with you.

13. When I say, "I'm doing okay," I wish you could understand that I don't "feel" okay and that I struggle daily.

14. I wish you knew that all of the grief reactions I'm having are very normal. Depression, anger,

hopelessness and overwhelming sadness are all to be expected. So please excuse me when I'm quiet and withdrawn or irritable and cranky.

15. Your advice to "take one day at a time" is excellent advice. However, a day is too much and too fast for me right now. I wish you could understand that I'm doing good to handle an hour at a time.

16. Please excuse me if I seem rude, it is certainly not my intent. Sometimes the world around me goes too fast and I need to get off. When I walk away, I wish you would let me find a quiet place to spend time alone.

17. I wish you understood that grief changes people. When my child (children) died, a big part of me died with them. I am not the same person I was before my children died, and I will never be that person again.

18. I wish very much that you could understand; my loss and my grief, my silence and my tears, my void and my pain. But I hope daily that you will never understand.

BRUCH: I simply tell people that I like to talk about my sons. They are a part of my family, but in a different way. If they are uncomfortable, they need to speak up, otherwise, I will continue to talk. I am not going to sit by and let my pain be bottled up. Ask any doctor; that is just not healthy to do. This has gotten me in trouble at work, but after what I went through, I just don't care. They don't even allow me pictures of my sons.

Even two years after their birthday, I still have flashbacks. I just recently remembered that my brother in-law, Matthew Scheller, carried my sons' casket. Only after talking to my husband did I find out that one of his friends, Scott Bauder, also carried them. I wish I could remember better; I feel that not only am I missing out on their lives, but the only few memories that I have are incomplete. We never took pictures of the service. It sounds so strange, but I wish I had. I can't remember the flowers, or the people who had come to celebrate their life. I have to realize that if I don't start to remember soon, I'll never remember. I was diagnosed with post-traumatic stress disorder four months after the twins' birth. I have changed, and will never be the same ever again.

MARTIN: BREATHE!!! Breathe and pray. Find support, do research, spread the word. I feel as if it's my responsibility to tell everyone that I know is having multiples about the possible dangers. Be positive, but plan for the worst. Miracles do happen. Look for the best care. I know what it feels like, but there is no comparison from one person to another. Everyone has different feelings, reactions, and situations. No one person knows it all, but know that you're not alone.

SLICHTER: Life is hard. It is a steep, slippery mountain that you have to climb without any ropes. Although there are hard times, there are many good times, too. Dealing with TTTS is one of those hard times. I wish that no one ever had to feel the way I did when I went through it. Sometimes things happen that we really have no control over, so deal with them one day at a time. Sometimes there will be good days, and sometimes there will be bad days. Don't be alone in this hard time, have a good support system. You will get through anything that life throws at you! The only thing you can do is keep your head high and your hopes higher.

DICK: Losing a child is devastating and many of us just want to crawl into a hole when it happens. The truth is, it's better to surround yourself with supportive people. They may not understand completely, but care enough about you to help you through the loss. You will need them.

Celebrate your children's lives, no matter how short. My husband and I celebrate our girls' birthday each year. The first year, we went to the river to be alone and think about them. We talked about them, and discussed how our lives were affected. It really helped to connect with each other. On the girls' second birthday, we went to the lake with our son and daughter and released balloons with hand written letters to our girls. This year, we're thinking of doing the same thing.

LIGHT: Stay strong, and do everything your doctor tells you to. Ask someone to help out as often as possible, so you can rest and let the babies grow! Eat well, drink Boost or Ensure every day, and stay positive. A lot of people may have negative comments, but believe in yourself and your babies, and don't listen to those people! I will never be able to put TTTS behind me. I will never forget our struggle because I'm faced with families going through it, other moms and TTTS survivor. We feel so blessed to have had such a great outcome after such a devastating disease. We're still working on how to explain their growth discordance; what will we say when they ask? What if they're too young to understand all the medical jargon? We'll find a way, I'm sure.

CHRISTMAN-SCHARER: My number one suggestion is to try to get a picture of your twins together. Whether they are alive, passed away, or one alive and one gone, take as many pictures of them as you can. We only have two of Karlyn alive, and they are not the greatest pictures. We have many of her after she passed away. Hold your babies. Even if they pass away, hold them. You will regret it if you don't.

Don't let other peoples' insensitivities get you. They don't know what you are going through, so don't try to make them. You will change. The "you" that you know will be gone, and another version of you will exist. After the loss of a child, things will never be the same. You will always miss them, and go through the "what ifs" every day.

MORGAN: Stay off your feet as much as possible, fill up on protein shakes/drinks, and try to refrain from using your stomach muscles (due to PROM). Get in contact with a TTTS support group to get as much information as you can about the disease.

REBILAS: I am a member of our local twins club, and known as the TTTS mom. I told them if someone is diagnosed, have them contact me. I have gone through it and am happy to share what I know. I also have two survivors, so that makes it a little less scary. I tell moms to do what I did: Bed rest! Ensure! And Dr. D! That isn't a guarantee, but it benefits the babies, and gives you something to focus on that you can control.

I also suggest contacting the foundation website. Mary, the founder, was such a wonderful aide during our pregnancy. We were so thankful for her, and for all she has done with the foundation. I offer to pray for any family, and am willing to take a phone call, anytime, just to talk, vent, or cry.

BENNER: I have only one regret; the internet scared me, so when I was first diagnosed, I didn't do much research. I would definitely recommend trying Boost and bed rest, as well as contacting other mothers who have been through it. Don't be scared.

HOPE: Every situation is different, so it is really hard to offer advice. I guess all I can say is get lots of rest, both mind and body! If anyone offers help, take it, the more support and help you have, the better you will be able to concentrate and cope with what is happening. Most of all, stay informed. Research what you don't understand, and learn as much as you possibly can.

WRIGHT: I would definitely start bed rest and protein shakes as soon as possible. Weekly ultrasounds are also a must, since so much can change in just one week. If one twin passes and you have a surviving twin, make any arrangements for burial, cremation, or memorial service, before the delivery. I am thankful that I didn't have to arrange everything while I had a newborn with medical needs. I had to stay pregnant with both of my girls for 19 weeks after Sarah died, in order to give Julie Anne the best chance at survival. Even though her body had decomposed some, I am forever grateful that I held her. I have no regrets in regards to my daughters and the TTTS. Even though I did lose Sarah, I'm glad that I didn't choose to terminate either of my babies. There are no "what ifs". I know that her death was what was supposed to happen.

BRAY: Keep your child's memory with you.

DILLE: The advice that I would give to a newly diagnosed TTTS parent would be to research all your options carefully and discuss them with a doctor whom you trust. Go with the option that is best for you and your pregnancy. Making that choice is sometimes very difficult to do. I felt surgery was the best option for us to save both babies. Even though we ended up losing Tessa, I know that we made the right choice for us. My heart still feels guilty, though. I'm hoping someday that will change.

The other advice I would give is to build a support system, and do it quickly. It could be family and friends, or it could be new people, online, who have dealt with TTTS. You will need support no matter where your TTTS journey takes you. And finally, love your babies! Don't be afraid to get too attached for fear of losing one or both of them. They need your love and support!

OROSZ: Be strong. Do your own research on the disease. Get in touch with Mary from the TTTS foundation. Share your feelings and don't be afraid to speak up. Never let the doctors tell you there isn't anything they can do, there is always something! Weigh all options, and remember, you can always find a different doctor.

FLETCHER: To any other parents going through TTTS, I would say take it one day at a time. Just pray,

pray, pray and know that you are not alone. I know that was the hardest part for me, thinking I was alone. Go through all the emotions. Keep good people around you, people who understand you, because you are going to have days where you can talk about it and days where you don't want to talk at all. There are a lot of wonderful groups out there for TTTS; I know it helped me to talk to people who had been through it. There are all kinds of information on the internet; it's a valuable resource. If you ever need to talk, I am always here for you, and so are all of the other moms. Though it may seem like you are never going to get through it, you will. God does answer prayers and he still performs miracles. There are wonderful doctors out there, too.

WALLINGTON: Stay strong and have faith. Do all you can to help your babies. Be your children's advocate. Get second opinions if you feel you need to. Educate yourself about TTTS and educate others. Lastly, be a voice. There are so many people with the disease, but sadly, some physicians do not know what TTTS is. By educating just one person, you could be saving a child's life. I will end this with my favorite quote, which I referred to in many times of weakness, "If God sends us on strong paths, we are provided strong shoes."

BRUCE: You should feel completely comfortable with your doctor and any decisions that your doctor makes. Remember, these are your children. If you don't like a doctor, or they are not answering your questions, go find a doctor who will. I didn't feel comfortable with my Maternal Fetal Medicine doctor from day one, but I didn't try to find another, nor did

I ask my OB to recommend another. It is a major "what if?"

If you have the heartbreaking experience of losing one or more of your children, do what feels right to you. Again, these are your children. If you want to take pictures, have a funeral, and light candles on the anniversary, then do it. Do not let others influence you against anything you want to do in honor and memory of your children. As a parent of a TTTS Angel, I know that a goodbye cannot be accomplished without a hello.

37
Moving on

BRUCH: It took me over 13 weeks to fully realize the emotional toll TTTS took. I didn't go back to work until after my due date. Every day was a challenge, my emotions never went away. I just learned how to cope with them better as time went on. Thankfully, the NICU made molds of Vincent's hands and feet. Ironically, between the days they passed, the hospital cut funds and changed from molds to impressions. I have only one foot and hand impression of Thomas. Please don't get me wrong, I love having something of them, but it hurts so much to not have identical mementos of my identical boys.

My husband still talks about them. We understand that we are still grieving, and we miss them on a daily basis. We have also acknowledged that I grieved differently than he has.

Seven months later, we found out we were going to have another baby. It was a singleton, and she was born healthy at 36 weeks. Since they had done a classical c-section for the twins, the doctors took her early, for fear that my uterus would rupture. The doctor had to make a different incision to get my daughter out. The twins' incision site had become paper thin, so had I had a big contraction, I would have ruptured and bled out. Though the doctor could not cut there, he did a great job. It was very scary, but he saved my life.

I will never completely "move on"; I am learning that if that is what I need to live my life, then so be it. In talking to moms, I have discovered that, from what I have seen, the rate of divorce after the loss of a child is around 85%, but only 10-15% of those will say that the death of the child caused them to break up.

SLICHTER: After the first year, my husband deployed to Iraq for 13 months. I went home to Texas and spent time with my family, where life became better. I was beginning to be happy again, and I could tell that my husband was, too. I think we just needed a change, and we got it. I got to spend time with my nephew, and life seemed to get back to normal. I got a job at a church nursery, taking care of babies on Sunday and Wednesday nights. I loved it so much. I have always loved kids.

Not a day goes by that I don't think of them, and sometimes I still cry, I miss them so much. I look at their pictures in their memory book, at the little tiny gown they put Jake in. I hold the blanket that they were wrapped in. I am so thankful that I had them in my life, even if they were only here for a few short months. They have taught me so much about myself, about life, but mostly about love - the never ending love that a parent has for a child. They have made me a stronger person; the woman I am today is because of them. They might not be alive now, but they are very alive in my heart, in my thoughts, and in my words.

CADLE: It has been a few years and I still have a hard time getting through, though it's not as devastating. My goal in life is to make sure that nobody ever makes the choice we did, to not hold our children. We were in such shock, which I can only assume was the reason. Ronnie looked at them briefly, but it was not enough. I pray at night for God to let me to see their faces, so that I might know what they look like, but He has not granted it yet. I know we will meet again one day and that they are with another brother or sister that we lost to an ectopic three months later.

The ectopic had ended April 12 2006, when I started bleeding and went to the hospital. I had emergency laser surgery to remove the pregnancy from my left ovary. Once again, I had lost a baby. I almost said, "That's it, I'm done, no more," but I prayed and relaxed, and in June 2006, we were pregnant again. On February 5, 2007, we had a 4 pound 11 oz. 17 1/2 inch long little girl - Isabella Grace Cadle!

MARTIN: It's hard to deal with the pain. My husband and I both grieve, but differently. I'm still not over my grandpa, who died in 07, nor my great grandmother, who passed in 01. My husband is not over the grandmother that raised him, who passed in 05. Today, we have each other. The boys are cared for and loved, up in heaven. They are our daughter's angels. The days, and life, go on. We don't know what else to do.

DICK: I think "moving on" isn't the right phrase. I will never be able to "move on" from the loss of my girls, but I am able to cope with it better each and every day. I have a 10 month old baby girl now; I look back and think, "If my girls had made it, I'd have three baby girls under the age of 3!" I'm also pregnant again. I'm not sure what I'm having, and frankly, I couldn't care less. I just want a healthy baby.

My son remembers his baby sisters, though he was only 3 when they were born. He loves to look at their gowns, and feet and hand prints, and to this day he will tell you, "I have three baby sisters, only two are in heaven." He's 6 now, and although he doesn't really understand what happened to them, he knows they're not here and misses them. I don't think the pain of losing a child ever goes away; I think we just learn to deal with it better as time goes on. RIP my baby angels, mommy loves you, her Brookelynn and Jazmen.

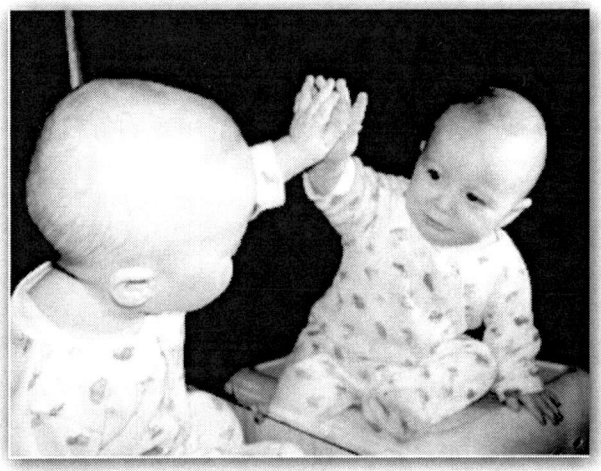

TUMMERS: Over time, we've dealt with our grief in our own way. Never does a day go by that I don't think of Cole, but many go by without tears. The biggest tears seem to come when Cameron is amazingly sweet, lovable and fun… it hurts so much then and seems so very unfair. I've never gone to counseling, except just after we lost him, but I spend a lot of time on the internet, talking to other TTTS moms and blogging about my grief. Writing helps a lot. Helping other moms, even those who didn't lose a twin, is very therapeutic. I was even honored to have helped a mom from England, who was touched and inspired by our story, and found such strength in my support, that she named her donor after Cole. I have always felt that God placed this journey in my life for a reason, and times like that make the reason pretty clear.

The biggest hurdle for me to overcome, even more than a year later, is guilt. I hate that I wasn't overjoyed at the news of twins, that I spent more time worrying about how we'd make it work than on thinking about the absolute miracles growing inside of me. I know now that it was how an organizer like me copes with stress but that doesn't stop me from sometimes thinking I wished this horrible thing upon myself. Thankfully, most days are much more positive, filled with the joy that is Cameron, and the wonderful gifts that being the mom of twins, even when one lives in Heaven, has given me.

My husband doesn't really talk about Cole a lot. When I am upset, he is great and comforts me, but it doesn't seem to affect him the same way. On Cole's angel day, we sent sky lanterns up to Heaven. Geoff was very upset that day. We talked a lot then, about our memories.

I thought their birthday might be a difficult day, and although it had moments, it really wasn't too bad. I wished I were celebrating with two babies, but I try each and every day to remind myself that I am blessed with one little miracle here, and one above. They have each taught me more in their short lives than I could ever have learned on my own.

CHRISTMAN-SCHARER: I had four other children to take care of, so I put all my effort into them. Don't get me wrong, it was hard; the first year is the hardest. It does get easier with time, but you will always think of your baby in heaven.

You will have the "what if's". You will experience all of the grieving stages, but some will last longer than others. Because Kylie survived, I know what Karlyn looks like, but that can be two-sided. You miss them more because can imagine having two babies that look alike. You wonder about their personality. It has been almost four years, and I go through this all the time. The kids miss her, too. We have a memory box of Karlyn's things, which my two younger kids love to look at, but Karl and the two older boys do not. We have her picture up with all the other kids; the sad thing is, as we update the other children's pictures, hers will always stay the same.

MORGAN: I have not yet been able to put TTTS behind me. Maybe it's because I stay at home with my son, and have a little more time to reflect. I am with Jadon day in and day out. When he is playing, I often imagine another little boy playing beside him. I catch myself fantasizing about two little boys running around my house. I have endured a lot of heartache by staying at home, but I feel glad and lucky for this opportunity to be with my son.

There isn't a day that goes by that I don't think about my other son. It's hard not to; Jadon is the spitting image of what his brother would have looked like. When Jadon gets to the age where he wants to celebrate or remember his brother, we will do so. He will be turning 3 this summer. I have not yet explained to him what happened, as he is too young to understand. However, he does know his brother's name. We plan to tell Jadon about the death of his brother when he gets older. My husband and I hope that he will continue to be a strong, happy, active person.

REBILAS: As I write this, I have two very healthy 5 year olds. We know how extremely blessed we are for our miracle boys! I assure other moms that they are just as sweet as little boys should be, with just the right amount of rotten-ness to make them adorable. The disease and NICU didn't slow them down one bit! We have moved on by helping where we can. Our boys had a few delays, but nothing that wasn't within a normal range. Our donor still weighs about 25% less than our recipient, but that doesn't stop him. As for walking, our recipient walked at 16 months and our donor at 19 months.

BENNER: There isn't a day that goes by that I don't think of them. I always wonder what they would look like, and if there was anything I could have done to save them. But there wasn't; I cannot blame my-self. To this day, I am still struggling with questions: "Why this?", "Why us?", and "What didn't we do?" Jacob and I believe that everything happens for a rea-son. Some days it's harder for me to accept that.

HOPE: For a while, I was very bitter about what we went through and the lack of support and under-standing we had. It took a while to realize I just had to let go.

I take every opportunity I can to talk about what we went through, to tell the stories of others who have suffered from TTTS, and to educate on the dangers of this syndrome. TTTS will always be in my life, not only through the memory of our experience, but through meeting and talking to people who have had to deal with it as well. It is a cause I will support for the rest of my life. I think everyone has something close to their heart, whether it is cancer research, heart disease, or something else. Although these causes are all extremely important, the most important one to me will always be TTTS.

Chloe and Jorja know the basic reason why they are different sizes, and as I wrote this, I read it to them chapter by chapter. Some things they understand, others they don't, but one thing is for sure: as time goes on, I know they will understand completely the seriousness of this syndrome, and how lucky they are to be here.

WRIGHT: I am still trying to move on. My daughters were delivered in October of 2009. I honestly feel like I lost a year of my life, with all the worry and fear for my daughters. We remember Sarah all the time. I never want Julie Anne to forget that she is a twin. I am proud to be a twin, and I want her to be, too. I will definitely tell my daughter all about my pregnancy, and everything that happened.

DILLE: If I am going to be completely honest, I would have to say that I have not put TTTS completely behind me. It is definitely a work in progress, but I'm not sure it will ever happen. It has been a little over 18 months since our diagnosis and loss. That time has helped heal the wounds some, but I believe this to be a wound that will never fully heal. As I mentioned before, I have a lot of guilt regarding the loss of Tessa. Maybe I didn't make the right choices, or maybe I could have done something different. This is the biggest issue that I still need to work through, to continue moving forward with my life. I am trying to do that by focusing on my beautiful, strong, happy, loving survivor, as well as my older children. I try to be positive, but some days are harder than others. It is still very difficult for me to see twins anywhere. Sometimes I can handle it okay, but most days I am filled with anger or sadness and just break down and cry. I say to myself over and over again, "I just want my baby girl back!"

We celebrate Tessa on anniversaries, birthdays, and holidays. My older children help pick out flowers, balloons and sometimes a small gift to take to Tessa. We write messages on some of the balloons, and send them up to the Heavens for Tessa to see. We talk to her and blow kisses to her, too. She is in our thoughts and prayers daily, always loved, never forgotten.

When the time is right, we will tell Cara about our TTTS journey, and about her beautiful identical twin sister, Tessa. I want Cara to know exactly who she is. I took pictures of the two of them together after birth, so that I could show Cara when she is old enough to handle seeing them. I have a feeling that Cara will know there is something missing in her life, even before we tell her about Tessa. Maybe, after we tell her, life will make more sense to her. I love my baby girls more than words can say, and hope that someday we will all be together again.

BRAY: I don't think I will ever be able to put TTTS behind me. I live in the UK, and at present, there is no official TTTS charity in operation. 85% of my research was done on American websites. My aim is to one day start my own charity, in memory of Oliver, and in honor of Thomas. I would love to create a foundation similar to the American TTTS Foundation.

We will always celebrate and remember our angel, Oliver. This year on the twins' birthday, we sent several sky lanterns with personal messages from the family on them. Then, on his angel day, we spent an evening at the beach, and let go 35 colorful balloons. Oliver is always very close to our hearts and we will always remember him. It is important to us, as a family, that we make his anniversaries very special. Thomas will always know about his TTTS journey; I talk about Oliver to all my children and he is a very big part of our family.

OROSZ: I have not put TTTS behind me, and never will. It will always be a part of our lives. Every time I look at my boys, I am still in shock that they are even here with us! They are my miracles!!

I want to share that CHOP mailed me the review of my placenta; they said the division was 60/40, and the cord insertion for Baby b (donor) was at the edge of the placenta. Although the share was 60/40, it didn't affect their growth.

When they are older, we will visit CHOP, and they will know of the trials we all went through to get them here. I am currently trying to get an article in the paper about my twins and TTTS. While I have been unsuccessful so far, I think it's mainly because I live in a small are, and the fact that TTTS isn't a well-known disease.

It breaks my heart every time I visit the TTTS Foundation's Facebook page and read peoples' stories. I hope they find what causes the disease and can save more lives. I also hope more doctors become familiar with the disease. Because my first doctor was not familiar with the disease, had I not switched doctors when I did, we might have lost our boys. That scares me tremendously.

<u>FLETCHER:</u> I don't think you ever move on. I think you just go numb and take it day by day. A death is hard to overcome, but when it is your child, the one you were supposed to protect, you are never the same again. It is always on your mind, and I think it gets harder every day. I try to get out and live my life, but it isn't easy when you feel like you are living a lie. Everyone handles every situation differently. You will find what works best for you, what helps you move on. I don't think I ever will, until I am in heaven with Abby.

I love all of my kids so much. Austin and Ally help me get through the day. They know when I need to laugh, when I need a smile, hug or kiss. I have some amazing kids.

Don't listen to people who don't know what they are talking about. Talk to people who have been through it; they won't judge you. They will listen and share, and you will know that it is ok to feel the way you do. There is nothing wrong with your emotions, or your guilt.

<u>DOBBS:</u> Today, the girls attend preschool at St. Francis Xavier Grade School. Ashlee plays softball and loves to swim. Emilee quit softball because it gives her a fever, but loves to ride her bike. The experience with TTTS changed our family forever, and we pray every day for those who make it and those who don't. It is a true miracle that they are both with us, and we thank God every day.

<u>BRUCE:</u> Moving on is sometimes difficult because TTTS parents who have lost try so hard to hang on. I have lost, but I have learned that you can move on yet still hang on. I reach out to other TTTS families,

spread awareness, and volunteer at a nearby NICU. I spend as much time as possible with my living children and husband. At first, moving on seems impossible. I thought it was never going to happen. The grief is stronger than I had ever imagined, but I know now that grief is what one makes of it. You can choose to let grief make you a better person, or you can let it make you a bitter person. I'd like to think that it has made me a better person, and that my children are proud of me.

38
Our Scenarios and Outcomes

Here is a quick reference of our treatment choices, scenarios, and outcomes:

Nothing was done or very little could be done:

Saved Both: Dobbs

Saved One: Bruce, Fletcher (membrane separated), Jelley (triplets, lost two)

Saved None: Dick, Cadle (triplets)

Amnio reductions w/o laser surgery:
Saved both and both lived for more than 1 year: Rebilas

Saved both and one lived for more than 1 year: Christman-Scharer

Saved both and both did not live for more than 1 year : Bruch

Amnio reduction w/ laser surgery:
Saved both and both lived for more than 1 year: Light, Hope, Orosz

Saved both and one lived for more than 1 year : Haddigan , Dille, Bray

Saved both from procedure and did not live for more than 1 year : Martin

Saved one and one lived for more than 1 year : Morgan

Lost both in utero after the procedure: Wright

Laser surgery w/o an amnio reduction (Septostomy):

Saved both and one lived for more than 1 year:
Tummers

Selection:

Saved none: SLICHTER (unable to complete selection
due to death of one baby)

39
Final Words

As you have read, every one of us had a completely different experience. Though similarities can be detected, each complete journey was their own. Each and every one of our lives will never be the same again. Whether or not our children came home with us, we still love them. Our hearts are with our children, no matter where they are.

We are all bonded for life, a kind of fraternity or club. We did not choose this in any way, shape, or form. We all wanted our babies. We all wanted to bring them home, and hoped to be woken up in the middle of the night hearing them cry. Unfortunately our husbands arc the ones waking up, hearing their wives cry. But some parents are fortunate. Their child or children survived the disease. In a different way, the survivors will be struggling with TTTS for all of their lives.

People keep telling me "things happen for a reason", but what purpose is there for an infant's death? In my case, our dreams were crushed. I will never know what they would be like, never heard them say "mommy," never looked into their eyes. I hate it when people say, "It happened for a reason".

There are some interesting statistics about what happens to a couple after they go through situations such as fertility treatment, or the death of a loved one. Here are some facts that are very important. I learned them in the support group I joined, after I lost my own twins:

1) 2/3 of all identical twin conceptions are Monochorionic - or fetuses that share one placenta
2) 98% of TTTS cases that go unchecked result in the loss of one or both fetuses
3) Here in the USA, the infant mortality rate is 630 per 100,000
4) 1 in 4 families experience a pregnancy loss

My boys never received regular birth certificates, or Social Security numbers. The only proof I have that they were even born is death certificates. Before this, I never knew how common infant death was. My boys were victims of a disease that kills, but there is hope that something can be done going forward. In a few years, when the camera used in fetoscopic laser photocoagulation surgery has been redesigned, we will see more survivors. However, if no one but those who have fought this disease take up the cause, then nothing more will be done. We must learn all we can from those that have come before, to help those who have yet to fight. We need to band together, look at the hard facts, and be willing to hear our mothers and women cry. We need to create a plan of action. The cost of sitting around and doing nothing is unimaginable. The pain that parents will experience is the worst pain of all. A parent should never have to bury their child, no matter what age or circumstance.

I hope that you have learned from this book. Every parent who has endured TTTS, no matter the outcome, wants a solution found, a cure, so that no more innocent children will suffer. Please join us in spreading the word and informing more people.

Thank you , Erin Bruch.

Contributors

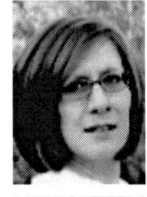 **Alicia Haddigan**

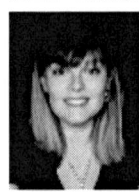 **Alison Morgan**

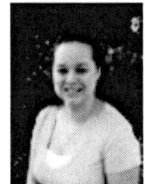 **Amanda Brenner**

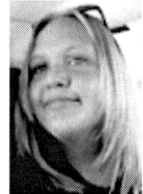 **Amanda Slichter**

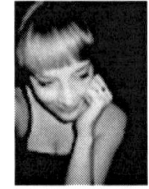 **Anne Marie Light**

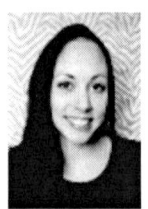 **Ashley Orosz**

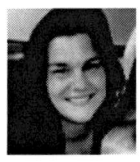 Bethany Wright

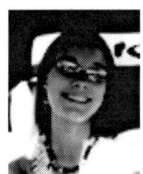 Courteney Dick

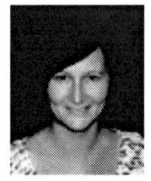 Emily Cadle

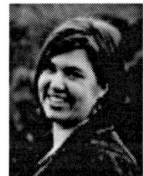 Erin Bruch

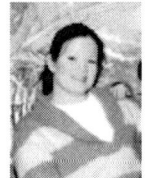 Holly Bruce

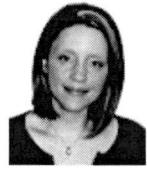 Jessica Dille

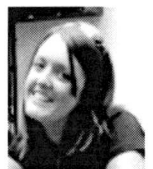 Joanne Bray

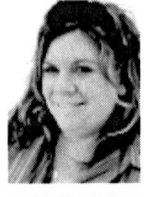 Jodie Tummers

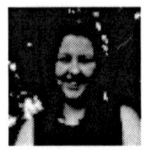 Melissa Hope

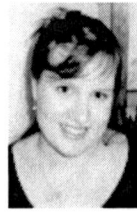 Mishael Jelley

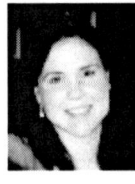 Rebecca Rebilas

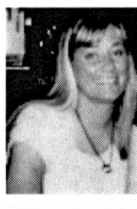 Robin Wallington

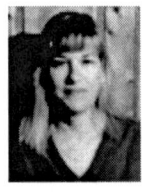 Shelley Christman-Scharer

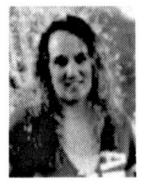 Stephanie Dobbs

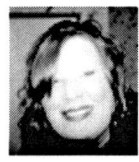 **Tonya Fletcher**

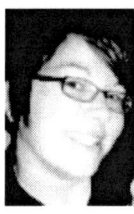 **Traci Martin**

Front Cover by Alisha Garrett Robertson

Illustrations by Jason Whymark

Back Cover by Melissa Hope

CPSIA information can be obtained at www.ICGtesting.com
Printed in the USA
BVOW061814101211

278071BV00006B/45/P